Medicare / Medigap

Medicare/Medigap

The Essential Guide for Older Americans and Their Families

HARRY SNYDER, CARL OSHIRO,

and the Editors of Consumer Reports Books

CONSUMERS UNION · Mount Vernon, New York

Library of Congress Cataloging-in-Publication Data
Medicare/Medigap : the essential guide for older Americans and their
   families / Harry Snyder, Carl Oshiro, and the editors of Consumer
Reports Books.
        p.   cm.
     Includes bibliographical references and index.
     ISBN 0-89043-412-3. — ISBN 0-89043-329-1 (pbk.)
     1. Medicare.   2. Medigap.   3. Aged—Medical care—United States.
4. Consumer education—United States.   I. Snyder, Harry.
II. Oshiro, Carl.   III. Consumer Reports Books.
RA395.A3M443   1990
368.4'26'00973—dc20

                                                              90-2020
                                                                CIP
                                                                Rev.

Second printing, February 1991
Manufactured in the United States of America

Medicare/Medigap is a Consumer Reports Book published by Consumers Union, the non-profit organization that publishes *Consumer Reports,* the monthly magazine of test reports, product Ratings, and buying guidance. Established in 1936, Consumers Union is char-tered under the Not-for-Profit Corporation Law of the State of New York.

Contents

Acknowledgments

We want to thank Judith Bell for the idea to write and produce this book. We also want to thank Bonnie Burns, Trudy Lieberman, Gail Shearer, and Peter Pipe for their contributions and help in the production of this book. The Health Care Finance Administration provided valuable technical assistance. We're also grateful to Sarah Uman, Chris Kuppig, and Roz Siegel of Consumer Reports Books for their confidence and encouragement.

Medicare / Medigap

Introduction

For the past ten years, much of our work as consumer advocates for the West Coast Regional Office of Consumers Union has been centered on health insurance and problems that seniors face in obtaining policies to supplement their Medicare coverage.

Through our contacts with seniors, we became aware of the problems that many have in understanding and utilizing the Medicare system. Confused by bills, forms, and unfamiliar terminology, many seniors are not getting the benefits they are entitled to by law. Still others are frightened by unethical salesmen into buying worthless or overlapping policies that they are told will cover what Medicare does not. We decided to write this book to provide answers to the questions about Medicare and supplemental policies we are so often asked.

Medicare's goal is to provide adequate health care and economic salvation for older Americans. Yet we hear more complaints than applause when people talk about Medicare. Many people are frightened and angry that not all costs of required health care may be paid. Some are confused about how to sign up for coverage and the difference between Hospital Insurance (Part A) and Medical Insurance (Part B) coverage. There can be frustration over the forms that have to be handled to keep track of payments and reimbursements. *Medicare/Medigap* will show you how to protect your health and your pocketbook with Medicare

1

and, if necessary, a private insurance policy to supplement Medicare coverage. In almost all cases, it's a simple, straightforward matter to sign up for Medicare and receive your benefits. Just sit down with this book and you will learn the simple steps to help you obtain the medical help needed to live a healthy, active, and productive life.

This easy-to-understand guide will also help you fill the gaps in Medicare coverage, assuring that you buy only what you need and really want while showing you how to avoid the hard-sell operators who prey on seniors' fears of catastrophic illness.

While Medicare does provide an essential service, aspects of the program, particularly provisions covering long-term care, need improvement. If you want to get involved and work with others to make the Medicare system work better or provide expanded coverage, *Medicare/Medigap* will show you how. Like Social Security, Medicare is heavily subsidized, with Medicare beneficiaries paying only a portion of the total cost. The best way to expand Medicare coverage is by making it a part of an overall plan for every American, old and young alike, to have comprehensive medical insurance.

Medicare/Medigap is written and arranged to be used as you need specific information. You do not need to sit down and read the whole book from cover to cover but can refer to a chapter when you want to learn about a specific issue or need to solve a particular Medicare problem. Of course, if you want to master all aspects of Medicare, it's here for you.

Either way, this book is a tool to make Medicare work for you. Use it in good health.

1

Medicare: What It Is and Who Is Eligible

Mrs. A is a 78-year-old widow with a mild heart condition. Three years ago, she fell down some stairs and broke her hip. Luckily, a neighbor saw her fall and came to help. Mrs. A was rushed by ambulance to the local hospital, where she was met by her family doctor. The doctor examined Mrs. A; then she admitted her to the hospital and arranged for a surgeon to repair her hip. She also called in a specialist to examine Mrs. A's heart. The specialist reported that her heart was fine, and the surgeon repaired her hip the following morning. Mrs. A stayed in the hospital for eight days.

She was then transferred to a skilled nursing home, where nurses and physical therapists helped her recuperate from the surgery. Mrs. A's doctor saw her several times in the hospital and continued to check on her condition in the nursing home. After 25 days, Mrs. A was well enough to go home.

Because sitting up and walking were still difficult for her, she needed a hospital bed and wheelchair during the first few months at home. Later, she was able to get around the house using a walker.

Three years later, Mrs. A has recovered from her fall. She walks without assistance and continues to live at home.

Mrs. A was fortunate. Most of her hospital and medical bills were paid for by Medicare, the health insurance plan for older Americans. Like millions of other seniors, Mrs. A could afford medical care because of the help of this government program.

Medicare was established by Congress in 1965 to help pay the cost of health care for senior citizens, certain younger disabled persons, and those with serious kidney disease. In 1989, the federal government spent about $100 billion for Medicare.

The cost of Medicare is shared by all Americans. Through payroll and income taxes, workers, employers, and other federal taxpayers who are not eligible for Medicare pay for about 90 percent of the cost of Medicare's hospital insurance program and for 75 percent of the cost of its medical insurance program. Medicare beneficiaries pay for the rest through regular premiums.

Over the years, the Medicare program has proven to be a far more efficient system for delivering benefits to the public than private insurance. While many improvements are needed in the program, 98 cents of every dollar spent by Medicare is for benefit payments, compared to only 60 cents of every dollar spent by private insurance companies.

Like private health insurance plans, Medicare pays for the services of doctors, hospitals, and other health-care providers that you choose, but it does not provide those services directly to you. Medicare operates no hospitals, nor does it hire any doctors, nurses, or others to care for patients. Its rules are set by the federal government, which hires private insurance companies to review Medicare claims and pay them.

Medicare now covers about 97 percent of those American residents over age 65. The program has two parts: Hospital Insurance (Part A) and Medical Insurance (Part B). Everyone who is receiving Social Security retirement benefits is automatically entitled to Part A coverage, but to receive Part B coverage, Medicare recipients must pay a monthly premium.

If you need to be hospitalized, Medicare Part A will cover the cost of most hospital services after you pay a certain set deductible charge. Medicare Part B helps pay for visits to doctors, outpatient hospital care, lab tests, X rays, and other services, as long as they are judged to be medically necessary. After you pay the first $75 of Medicare-covered medical expenses each year, Medicare pays 80 percent of whatever charges it has approved for the further medical services you receive in that year. In most cases, you are responsible for paying any charges that are not covered by Medicare or that are over the Medicare-approved amount.

Medicare is sometimes confused with another government program, Medicaid. Medicaid is designed to pay for health care for low-income people of all ages. To receive Medicaid benefits, your income and assets must fall below certain thresholds. Each state operates its own Medicaid program, and the thresholds and rules vary considerably.

In general, you are eligible for Medicaid if your annual income and assets (not including your home) are each less than $3,000. Most states also cover persons who are "medically needy"— people who have incomes above the Medicaid threshold but have particularly high medical expenses. When these expenses are subtracted from their incomes, they become financially needy enough to qualify for Medicaid.

In all states, Medicaid covers inpatient and outpatient hospital care, doctors' services, home health care, medical transportation, and lab and X-ray services. Unlike Medicare, Medicaid pays for custodial care, and in some states, it covers additional services such as prescription drugs and foot, dental, and eye care.

While Medicaid is not a medical assistance program designed specifically for the elderly, many of those covered by the program are above age 65. Because Medicare does not cover long-term custodial care, the only option for many seniors who need that care is to deplete their resources until they are poor enough to qualify for Medicaid. Currently, nearly one in five Medicaid recipients is elderly, and nearly 40 percent of all Medicaid funds go to elderly recipients. (See Chapter 11.)

WHO IS ELIGIBLE FOR MEDICARE?

Most people over 65 are entitled to Medicare Part A (Hospital Insurance) benefits because they are eligible for Social Security retirement benefits. You are also entitled to Medicare Part A if you are eligible for railroad retirement benefits. You do not have to pay anything to receive this Medicare coverage, but you do need to sign up for it. When you enroll in Part A, you will be automatically signed up for Part B (Medical Insurance), for which you will have to pay a monthly premium. This Part B premium was $28.60 per month in 1990. You can, however, refuse Part B coverage.

You are also entitled to receive Part A benefits if you are under 65 and have been eligible for Social Security disability benefits for at least 24 months. If you are already receiving disability benefits, you will be automatically enrolled in Part A and Part B, beginning with the 25th month. You will not be charged a monthly premium for Part A. Unless you refuse the Part B Medical Insurance, however, a Part B premium will be deducted from your monthly disability check. Medicare coverage will continue until you are no longer disabled.

If you are not receiving disability benefits but have a physical or mental impairment that prevents you from "any substantial gainful activity" for at least a year, check with your local Social Security office to find out whether you are entitled to those benefits.

If you are under age 65 and have a kidney impairment that "appears irreversible and permanent and requires a regular course of dialysis or kidney transplantation to maintain life," and you or your spouse qualify for Social Security or railroad retirement benefits, you are entitled to Part A.

For dialysis patients, coverage begins either one or three months after treatment begins, depending on whether the treatment occurs at home or in an institution. Coverage stops one year after the end of regular dialysis treatment. For kidney transplant patients, coverage may begin as early as the month in which you are hospitalized for the transplant and continues for three years. For more information, consult the booklet "Medicare Coverage for Kidney Dialysis and Kidney Transplant Services," available from your local Social Security office.

If you are over 65 and are not entitled to Part A, you can still receive Part A coverage by voluntarily enrolling in Medicare and paying a monthly premium. If you sign up voluntarily for Part A, you must also sign up for Part B. Voluntary enrollment is open to anyone over 65 who (1) is a resident of the United States, and (2) is either (a) a US citizen or (b) lawfully admitted as a permanent resident who has resided in the United States continuously for at least five years immediately preceding his or her application for coverage.

HOW AND WHEN TO SIGN UP

If you plan to retire at age 65, apply for your retirement benefits at your local Social Security office about three months before the date you actually retire. This will give the government plenty of time to process your application. You do not have to fill out a separate application for Medicare; you will be signed up for Hospital Insurance and Medical Insurance automatically when you apply for your retirement benefits. Your coverage will begin on the first day of the month in which you reach your 65th birthday.

If you plan to retire before you are 65, apply for your retirement benefits three months before the date you actually retire. No separate application is needed for Medicare. However, *Medicare coverage will not begin when you retire,* but on the first day of the month in which you have your 65th birthday. Unless your employer's health plan covers retirees, you will need to buy private insurance to cover you until Medicare coverage begins. The cost of that insurance is likely to be expensive.

If you plan to retire after you are 65 but want Medicare coverage to begin at 65, fill out Form HCFA 18-F5 at your local Social Security office. Your coverage will begin on the first day of the month that you turn 65. Again, it is a good idea to apply three months before your 65th birthday.

In addition to Medicare, you may be covered by a group health plan through your job if you keep working after you turn 65. Employers with 20 or more workers are required by federal law to give workers over 65 (and their spouses) the same health-care coverage that they give younger workers. If you or your spouse are working and are covered by both Medicare and an employer-sponsored group health plan, you may choose that plan to have primary responsibility for paying for covered services. Medicare will then pay only for services not covered by the employer-sponsored health insurance. (See Chapter 7.)

If you do not qualify for Social Security retirement benefits, you may still sign up for Medicare, but enrollment is possible only during certain periods. The first and best opportunity to sign up is during your initial enrollment period, which begins three months before the first day of the month in which you have your 65th birthday and extends for seven months. For example, if your 65th birthday is on August 25, 1990, your initial enrollment period begins on May 1, 1990, and ends on November 31, 1990.

If you do not enroll during the initial enrollment period, you may still sign up during any general enrollment period, an annual three-month window that runs from January 1 to March 31 each year. Be aware that you will have to pay a penalty if you do not sign up during your initial enrollment period, however. In general, the penalty is 10 percent, and the longer you delay, the bigger the penalty.

For Part A (Hospital Insurance), the premium is increased by 10 percent and remains in effect for twice the number of years that enrollment was delayed. For Part B (Medical Insurance), the premium is increased by 10 percent for each year that enrollment was delayed. For example, if you were 65 in 1988 but waited two years to enroll in both Hospital Insurance and Medical Insurance, each month you would pay the Hospital Insurance premium of $175 plus a late enrollment penalty of $17.60, as well as the Medical Insurance premium of $28.60 plus a penalty of $5.80. The Hospital Insurance penalty would be removed after four years.

If you continue to work after 65 and are covered by your employer's health plan, you can delay enrolling in Part B without any penalty. Simply sign up three months before you actually retire. Similar penalties apply if you sign up for Medicare, terminate your coverage, and later re-enroll.

The penalties are intended to discourage people from signing up for Medicare only when they become ill. Too many ill people at one time would cost so much that the program would be unable to pay for covered services.

PREMIUMS

If you are over 65, you will be required to pay a Hospital Insurance premium for Part A only if you do not qualify for Social Security or railroad retirement benefits. For those who voluntarily sign up for Medicare, the monthly premiums (in 1990) are $175 for Part A and $28.60 for Part B. If you qualify for Social Security or railroad retirement benefits, there is no premium for Part A, but you must pay the Part B premium unless you specifically refuse that coverage.

Both premiums are set each year according to a complex set of requirements established by Congress, and have increased each year because of the escalating cost of providing hospital and medical services.

If you are receiving Social Security or railroad retirement benefits, the Part B premium will be automatically deducted from your monthly benefit check. If you are not receiving these benefits, you must pay your premiums directly by a check or money order to a regional Social Security medical insurance center. You will be billed quarterly. Since these bills often arrive only a few days before they are due, be sure you are prepared to mail a check the day you receive the bill to keep your payments current. Write your name and Medicare claim number on all checks, and keep copies of all paid bills.

If your payment is late, there is a grace period before your coverage lapses, entending to the last day of the second month following the due date. For example, if a payment was due on January 1, the grace period extends to March 31. This initial grace period may be extended if the government finds that you had "good cause" for not paying the premium. If you were mentally or physically incapable of paying, or if you had good reason to believe that payment had been made, or if an administrative error occurred, you probably had "good cause." If you mail the payment on or before the last day of the grace period, coverage will continue without any interruption; if not, coverage will be terminated and you will be sent a notice of termination.

<u>YOUR MEDICARE CARD</u>

After you sign up for Medicare, you will receive your Medicare card in the mail. The card is proof that you are covered by the program. It contains the following important information:

1. *Your Medicare claim number.* This is your Social Security number with a letter and occasionally a number added. (Though the letter following your Social Security number is often an *A* or a *B*, it has no relationship to whether you have Part A or Part B coverage.) The claim number is your means of identification in the Medicare system. You should use it in all your claims and correspondence about Medicare coverage and benefits.

2. *Your coverage.* The card states whether you have Hospital Insurance (Part A), Medical Insurance (Part B), or both.

3. *The date your coverage began.* For each type of coverage, the card will give the date your coverage actually began. For most people who enroll in both Part A and Part B, this will be the same date.

When you receive your Medicare card (see Appendix C), review it to make sure that the information on it is correct. If you find an error, call Social Security. (You can find the number in your local telephone directory under U.S. Government, Department of Health and Human Services, Social Security Administration.) If the information is correct, sign the card and carry it in your wallet where you can find it easily. You will need to show

Send for Your Free Medicare Update

Since the laws governing Medicare costs and benefits change frequently, the authors of *Medicare/Medigap* have prepared an easy-to-read update that will provide you with up-to-the-minute information on this important topic. To order your free copy, please fill out the coupon below (or a facsimile) and return it along with a stamped, self-addressed business envelope to:

Medicare Update
Consumers Union
West Coast Regional Office
1535 Mission Street
San Francisco, CA 94103

Medicare Update

Name_____

Street Address_____ Apt._____

City_____ State_____ Zip_____

You must enclose a stamped, self-addressed business envelope and this coupon (or facsimile) to receive your free supplement.

the card when you go to a doctor, clinic, hospital, or other health-care provider. Some providers may want to copy the card so that they can bill Medicare correctly.

It's a good idea to make a copy of your Medicare card yourself in case the original is lost. Keep the copy where it is safe but easily retrievable. (See Chapter 13.)

If you lose your card, call or visit your local Social Security office. It generally takes about 45 days before you will receive your new card in the mail. If you know your Medicare identification number, you can continue to receive Medicare benefits while you are waiting. If you do not, your Social Security office can give you a temporary proof of Medicare coverage.

2

What Medicare Covers

PART A (HOSPITAL INSURANCE)

Medicare Hospital Insurance (Part A) covers expenses if you are admitted to a hospital, skilled nursing facility, or Christian Science sanatorium. It also covers some types of home health care and hospice care for terminally ill patients.

Inpatient Hospital Care

If you need to be hospitalized, Medicare Hospital Insurance will pay for

- a semi-private room (two to four beds to a room)
- all meals, including special diets
- regular nursing services
- special units (such as intensive care, coronary care, etc.)
- drugs supplied during the hospitalization
- lab tests
- blood transfusions
- X rays and other radiology services
- medical supplies (casts, dressings, splints, etc.)
- use of appliances such as wheelchairs
- operating room and recovery room costs
- rehabilitation services (physical therapy, occupational therapy, and speech pathology services)

Medicare will not cover charges for personal conveniences (television, telephones, etc.), private duty nurses, or a private room, unless judged medically necessary. Nor will it pay for services provided in a foreign hospital, except in certain extremely limited circumstances involving Canadian or Mexican hospitals. Services in a Canadian or Mexican hospital are covered only if

1. You are in the United States when an emergency occurs but the Canadian or Mexican hospital is closer than the nearest American hospital that can provide the needed emergency service, or

2. You live in the United States but the Canadian or Mexican hospital is closer to your home than the nearest U.S. hospital that can provide the needed care, or

3. You are traveling through Canada by the most direct route to or from Alaska and another state when an emergency occurs requiring that you be admitted to a Canadian hospital.

Part A pays benefits for inpatient hospital care for each "spell of illness." A spell of illness is counted from the first day you are admitted to a hospital and extends for a period of 60 days. A second spell does not begin until you have been out of the hospital (or other facility primarily providing skilled nursing or rehabilitation services) for 60 days and are then readmitted. If you are in the hospital for 40 days, return home for 10, and then have a relapse requiring further hospitalization, Medicare will consider you are in the 41st day of your first spell of illness.

For each spell of illness, you pay a deductible of $592 (in 1990). After that, Medicare will pay 100 percent of the cost of covered services for the first 60 days you are in the hospital. For days 61 through 90, you are responsible for $148 per day (in 1990); Medicare will pay the rest.

If you are hospitalized for longer than 90 days, you can claim up to 60 "reserve days." For each reserve day, Medicare will pay all of the cost of covered services except for $296 per day (in 1990). If you have one or more regular benefit days available when you enter the hospital, the entire bill will be paid under the Medicare Prospective Payment System, and you will not have to use your lifetime reserve days. Once you use a reserve day, however, it cannot be replaced. Each Medicare beneficiary has only 60 reserve days during his or her lifetime. Medicare will also pay for up to 190 days of inpatient care in a psychiatric hospital during your lifetime.

If you need a blood transfusion while you are a patient in a hospital, Medicare will cover the cost except for the charge for the first three pints. You can avoid this charge by either donating an equal amount of blood or arranging for someone to donate it for you.

While this coverage may not seem generous, it is usually adequate. About 20 percent of Medicare beneficiaries are admitted to a hospital each year, and the average hospital stay is about nine days. Fewer than one percent of Medicare beneficiaries are admitted to psychiatric hospitals, and their average stay is about 22 days.

Skilled Nursing Care

Medicare will pay for inpatient care in a skilled nursing home or rehabilitation center if the following conditions are met:

1. You were hospitalized for at least three consecutive days and transferred to a Medicare-certified skilled nursing facility within 30 days of leaving the hospital.

2. Your condition requires skilled nursing care or rehabilitation services that must be performed directly by or under the supervision of highly trained personnel.

3. Your condition requires these services on a daily basis.

4. As a practical matter, considering efficiency and economy, these services can only be provided on an inpatient basis in a skilled nursing facility.

These services must be provided under your doctor's orders, and he or she must periodically certify that all of these conditions continue to be satisfied. The services must be provided in a facility that meets minimum standards established by Medicare and that has agreed to accept Medicare patients.

If you qualify, Medicare will pay for up to 100 days of care per spell of illness. The services covered in a skilled nursing facility are similar to those covered in a hospital: semi-private room, skilled nursing care, rehabilitation services, inpatient drugs, blood, medical appliances, and so on. During the first 20 days, Medicare will pay 100 percent of the cost of covered services. For days 21 through 100, you are responsible for a co-payment of $74 per day.

Most senior citizens who need care in a nursing home, however, will not be able to satisfy these conditions—particularly the requirement for skilled nursing care, which must be provided by registered nurses, physical or occupational therapists, speech pathologists, or audiologists. Instead, most seniors who enter a nursing home need "custodial care"—help with dressing, bathing, eating, preparing meals, mobility, and other daily activities. Unfortunately, custodial care is not covered by Medicare. (See Chapters 10 and 11).

Care in Christian Science Sanatoria

Inpatient hospital care and skilled nursing care provided in Christian Science sanatoria are covered to the same extent as care provided in regular hospitals and skilled nursing facilities. The same deductible and co-payments apply. To qualify, the sanatoria must be operated or listed and certified by First Church of Christ Scientist, Boston, Massachusetts.

Home Health Care

Medicare will cover the cost of skilled nursing care, rehabilitation care, and other health-care services provided in your home under certain conditions. To qualify, you must be confined to your home and need some skilled nursing care or physical or speech therapy. You must be under a doctor's care, and the doctor must establish and periodically review a written plan of care that includes a program of home health care.

If these conditions are met, Medicare will pay for

- part-time or intermittent skilled nursing care
- physical, occupational, or speech therapy
- part-time or intermittent services of home health aides

"Part-time or intermittent" usually means for a few hours a day several times a week but may mean more or less, depending on individual circumstances. Medicare guidelines allow for daily care for five days a week for up to two or three weeks. Medicare will not pay for full-time care on a permanent or indefinite basis.

Covered services must be either provided or arranged by a home health agency certified by Medicare. (Your doctor should be able to refer you to some agencies that can provide the services you need.) The agency will bill Medicare directly for 100 percent of the cost of covered services. There are no deductibles or co-payments. By law, a home health agency is prohibited from billing you for any charges and must refund any money improperly collected.

Hospice Care

Hospice care is a special method of caring for patients who are terminally ill. Hospice programs care for patients in their homes whenever possible and emphasize relieving pain and managing symptoms rather than undertaking curative procedures. Medicare will pay for up to 210 days of hospice care if the following three conditions are met:

1. A doctor certifies that a patient is terminally ill.
2. The patient elects to receive care from a hospice instead of the standard medical benefits for the terminal illness.
3. Care is provided by a Medicare-certified hospice program.

If these conditions are met, Medicare will pay for

- nursing services
- doctors' services
- drugs, including outpatient drugs for pain relief and symptom management
- physical, occupational, and speech therapy
- home health aides and homemaker services
- medical social services
- medical supplies and appliances
- short-term inpatient care and inpatient respite care
- training and counseling for the patient and family members

After a patient decides in favor of hospice care, Medicare will not pay for treatments relating to the terminal illness other than for pain relief and symptom management. Standard Medicare benefits resume only if the patient revokes his choice.

Medicare pays in full for nearly all covered hospice services. The exceptions are that patients are responsible for the lesser of $5 or 5 percent of the cost of outpatient drugs, and for 5 percent of the cost of inpatient respite care (approximately $3 to $5 per day, depending on where the patient lives).

PART B (MEDICAL INSURANCE)

Medicare Medical Insurance (Part B) covers a wide range of medical expenses, including those for doctors' services, lab tests, outpatient hospital services, medical equipment, and supplies. In general, you pay the first $75 each year, after which Medicare pays for 80 percent of its approved charge for covered services. In most cases, you are still responsible for any excess charges beyond the Medicare-approved charges.

Doctors' Services

Medical Insurance (Part B) covers a doctor's services whether you receive the services in the doctor's office, a hospital, a nursing home, or your home. However, the services must be delivered in the United States. Though Medicare will pay for most doctors' services, Medicare will *not* pay for

- routine physical examinations
- routine foot care
- eye or hearing exams for prescribing eyeglasses or hearing aids
- routine immunizations
- cosmetic surgery (unless needed because of accidental injury, or to improve the function of a malformed part)

Under Part B, once you meet the $75 annual deductible, Medicare pays 80 percent of its "approved charge" for services provided by your doctor. Currently, Medicare establishes its approved charges based on the lesser of the doctor's "usual and customary charge" for a service, the "prevailing charge" in the community for that service, or the doctor's actual charge. Both the "usual and customary charge" and the "prevailing charge" are determined by complex formulas requiring hundreds of calculations. The procedure results in established, approved charges that vary from area to area. But be aware that with certain exceptions, in general, doctors are free to charge their Medicare patients amounts that are higher than the approved charge. In most cases you are responsible for paying those excess charges. Connecticut and Massachusetts have passed laws that prohibit doctors from charging Medicare patients more than the Medicare-approved amount. Rhode Island and Vermont prohibit doctors from imposing excess charges on low-income Medicare patients.

Doctors who agree to accept the charges approved by Medicare and not to impose any excess charges on their Medicare patients are said to accept "Medicare assignment." These doctors bill Medicare directly for covered services. Medicare pays them 80 percent of the approved charge less any part of the annual $75 deductible that has not been met. You pay the deductible and the other 20 percent of the approved charge. No other fees are collected for covered services.

There are several ways in which doctors accept assignment. Some doctors, known as participating physicians, sign a contract with Medicare agreeing to accept assignment for all services they provide to all Medicare patients. Other doctors accept assignment only for some patients but not for others. Some doctors are even more selective and accept assignment only for a particular service to a particular patient.

The number of doctors who accept Medicare assignment in a community varies widely. Nationwide, about 40 percent of all doctors accept assignment for all their Medicare patients. The rest may accept assignment only when they believe that the patient is unable to pay the extra charge. In Alabama, 76 percent of the doctors accept assignment, while in some states fewer than 20 percent do so. (See Appendix D.)

To find a doctor in your area who is a participating physician, consult the *Medicare Participating Physician/Supplier Directory*. You can obtain a copy by calling or writing the insurance company that handles your Medicare claims, or you can consult one at your local Social Security office. Some insurance companies will provide you over the phone with the names of local doctors who accept assignment. (To find the insurance company that handles your Medicare claims, see Appendix A.)

If you already have doctors whom you like, ask them if they will accept assignment for all their services once you enroll in Medicare. Many people feel uncomfortable discussing financial topics with doctors, but Medicare assignment can save you hundreds of dollars if you need to visit the doctor often. This is an important issue that most doctors are willing to discuss; many of them benefit substantially from treating Medicare patients.

Because your main interest when you are sick is in getting well, not in paying medical bills, you may find it easier to ask about assignment before you need medical attention. Some people find it more comfortable to discuss the subject over the phone instead of during a hurried office visit. If you feel uncomfortable discussing it yourself, ask someone you trust (a family member, friend, neighbor, insurance counselor, or the like) to talk to the doctor for you.

The current method of calculating what fees constitute approved charges for doctors is so complex that Congress has directed the Health Care Financing Administration to adopt a new method based on a more uniform schedule of fees. This new method will be phased in from 1992 to 1997. As part of this reform, beginning in 1992, doctors who do not accept assignment will be prohibited from charging fees that are more than 15 percent above the Medicare-approved amount.

Chiropractic Care

Medicare does not cover most chiropractic care. The only service covered is physical manipulation of the spine to correct a dislocation, misalignment, off-centering, fixation, or abnormal spacing of the spine that can be demonstrated by an X ray.

Foot Care

Medicare will not pay for routine care for flat feet, corns, calluses, etc. But care for some of these conditions may be covered when the care is necessary to the treatment of a separate medical condition. For example, ordinary corns, calluses, and blisters can cause serious medical problems for people with diabetes. Consequently, Medicare will pay for treatment of these conditions as part of the overall care for these patients.

Eye Care

Medicare pays for fitting of corrective lenses only if they are prosthetic lenses that replace the natural lens of the eye. It does not pay for routine eye exams or eyeglasses.

Dental Care

Medicare will pay only for dental care that involves: (1) surgery of the jaw or related structures, (2) setting fractures of the jaw or facial bones, or (3) services that would be covered if performed by a doctor. It does not cover routine care involving treatment, filling, or removal of teeth, or gum surgery. If a dental condition requires you to be hospitalized, Medicare Part A will cover the hospital expenses less the annual hospital deductible, even if none of the professional care is covered by Part B.

Ambulance Services

Medicare will pay for medically necessary ambulance service.

Durable Medical Equipment

Medicare will pay for the cost of buying or renting durable medical equipment such as wheelchairs and oxygen equipment, but all such equipment must be prescribed by your doctor. In general, equipment costing over $150 must be rented and not purchased if you expect Medicare to pay for it. If it costs less than $150, you may either rent or buy it. These rules change frequently, however, so check with the insurance company that handles your Medicare claims before buying or renting any equipment.

Blood Transfusions

If you need a blood transfusion but are not a hospital inpatient, Part B will pay 80 percent of its approved charge after the first three pints in any calendar year. The three-pint deductible is separate from the three-pint deductible under Part A. To the extent the deductible is met under one part, it does not have to be met under the other.

Outpatient Hospital Services

Medicare will pay for 80 percent of the approved charge for outpatient hospital services, including care provided in an emergency room or outpatient clinic. You are responsible for the remaining 20 percent.

Outpatient Physical Therapy, Occupational Therapy, and Speech Pathology

Medicare will cover outpatient physical therapy, occupational therapy, and speech pathology services prescribed by your doctor. It will pay for 80 percent of the approved charge for these services if they are provided in an outpatient hospital facility, in a skilled nursing facility, or by a Medicare-certified rehabilitation agency or home health agency. You are responsible for the remaining 20 percent.

If these services are provided by an independently practicing, Medicare-certified physical or occupational therapist in the patient's home or therapist's office, Medicare will pay only up to $400 a year. The regular deductible and co-payment requirements also apply. Unless an independent therapist has agreed to accept assignment, he or she may bill you for excess charges. There is no coverage for services provided by an independently practicing speech pathologist.

Mental Health Services

Part B will pay for 80 percent of the cost of mental health services if the services are prescribed by your doctor and provided through a hospital outpatient program. This benefit is not subject to the 190-day limit under Part A for *inpatient* hospitalization for the treatment of mental illness. The services covered include diagnostic services, family counseling, psychiatric social services, and individual, group, or activity therapy. But there is a limit to how much Medicare will pay for doctors' services. Part B counts as covered expenses only 62.5 percent of its approved charges up to a maximum of about $1,400 each year for doctors' services for outpatient treatment of mental illness.

Clinical Laboratory Tests

In most cases, Medicare will pay the full cost of clinical laboratory tests. Clinical lab tests are tests done on body fluids such as blood or urine. Both independent labs and doctors must bill Medicare directly for 100 percent of the cost of covered lab services and cannot bill you for any deductibles, co-payments, or charges of any kind.

Medical Supplies

Medical supplies such as surgical dressings, splints, and casts ordered by your doctor to treat your condition are covered by Medicare, but routine first-aid supplies such as adhesive tape or antiseptics are not.

WHAT MEDICARE DOES NOT COVER

1. Some important services that are not covered by Medicare include custodial care, long-term home health care, routine physical exams, prescription drugs, and most kinds of routine eye, hearing, foot, and dental care.

2. You are also responsible for *deductibles*, amounts you have to pay for covered services before Medicare begins to pay. For example, if you were hospitalized in 1990, you were responsible for the first $592 in charges. That $592 is known as the hospital deductible. Medicare pays the remaining hospital expenses during the first 60 days that you are in the hospital.

3. For many services covered by Medicare, you have to contribute a *co-payment*. Under Part B, Medicare will pay only part of the approved charges (typically 80 percent), and you are responsible for the rest. For example, if you have a doctor's bill of $300 and Medicare's approved charges for those services are $300, Medicare will pay $240; you are responsible for the remaining $60. Your portion is called a co-payment, or co-insurance.

Under Part A, you are responsible for a 25 percent co-payment for the 61st day through the 90th day in a hospital and a 50 percent co-payment for each of the 60 reserve days if your stay is longer than 90 days. In a skilled nursing facility, you are also responsible for a co-payment of $74 for the 21st day through the 100th day.

4. You may also be responsible for *excess charges*. For many services covered by Part B, including doctors' services, Medicare calculates its payment based on an approved charge for the service provided. As we noted, the approved charge is often less than the actual amount charged. For example, your doctor may charge you $125 for a procedure when the Medicare-approved charge for that procedure is only $100. The $25 difference is an excess charge. In some instances, you are responsible for paying that difference in addition to any deductibles and co-payments that you owe. You can protect yourself against excess charges by finding a doctor who accepts Medicare assignment and will charge no more than the amounts approved. (See pages 18 to 20.) In 1992, the doctor will not be allowed to charge you more than $115 when the Medicare-approved charge is $100.

THE REPEAL OF CATASTROPHIC COVERAGE

In 1988 and 1989, Congress first overwhelmingly passed, then repealed, the Medicare Catastrophic Coverage Act. That law represented the single largest expansion of the Medicare program since it was established in 1966. The battle over the new law focused largely on who should pay for the cost of new Medicare benefits.

The Catastrophic Coverage Act of 1988 was intended to help older Americans with large hospital and medical bills by

1. paying for an unlimited number of days of hospitalization after an initial deductible

2. increasing the number of covered days of skilled nursing-home care and hospice care

3. paying for 100 percent of the approved cost of doctors' services after a beneficiary's Part-B co-payments and deductibles exceeded a catastrophic level (about $1,370 a year), and

4. paying half of the cost of prescription drugs for beneficiaries with large drug expenses

The new benefits would cost about $12 billion a year when fully implemented.

For the first time in Medicare's history, Congress required that Medicare beneficiaries pay the entire cost of the new benefits rather than imposing the cost on the general working population. About two-thirds of the cost of the catastrophic-care law was to be collected through a supplemental premium based on a beneficiary's income tax liability. The more taxable income beneficiaries had, the greater the supplemental premium they were required to pay, up to a maximum of $800. In any one year, only 36 to 43 percent of the persons eligible for Medicare would have paid any supplemental premium. One-third of the cost of the new benefits was to be collected from an increase in the Part B premium paid by all enrollees.

Even before the law was fully implemented, there were calls for repeal. Leading the attack were affluent older Americans who were angry about the higher supplemental premiums they were required to pay. Also pressing for repeal were seniors with supplemental insurance who believed that they already had protection against catastrophic expenses. As a result of their efforts, in 1989 Congress voted overwhelmingly to repeal the Catastrophic Coverage Act, nullifying both the expanded coverage and the new premiums it had passed only a year before.

The repeal was a victory for those seniors with the highest incomes, who would have paid the highest supplemental premiums. It was also a victory for insurance companies, which would now be able to sell more policies to seniors by emphasizing the gaps in Medicare coverage.

The losers in this process were the 60 to 70 percent of older Americans who would have received more in new benefits than they would have paid in new premiums. Hit hardest were those living on low or moderate incomes with no additional insurance to supplement Medicare coverage. For these seniors, the loss of the Catastrophic Coverage Act meant that they were no longer protected against large hospital and medical expenses.

Seniors who have Medicare supplement insurance may also have to pay more. What they saved in lower taxes may be more than eaten up by higher insurance premiums. A survey by the General Accounting Office found that insurance companies increased their monthly premiums for those "Medigap" policies by about 20 percent following the repeal of the Catastrophic Coverage Act.

3

Closing the Gaps in Medicare Coverage: A Survey of Additional Options

Because of the gaps in Medicare coverage, many seniors buy additional insurance to supplement Medicare. But not all seniors need supplemental insurance, and many who do need such insurance buy either too much or the wrong kind.

BUYING SUPPLEMENTAL INSURANCE

Nearly three out of four Americans on Medicare have some kind of supplemental health insurance. Some seniors already are covered through employer group plans that extend coverage to retirees. But most seniors on Medicare buy a Medicare supplement policy or some other kind of insurance from insurance agents, through groups, or directly from an insurance company by mail.

There are several different types of insurance sold to seniors. They include Medicare supplement policies (see Chapter 4), hospital indemnity insurance, medical-surgical policies, accident insurance, and cancer or dread-disease insurance, but only Medicare supplement policies are specifically designed to supplement Medicare.

MEDICARE SUPPLEMENT INSURANCE

Medicare supplement insurance (known colloquially as Medigap insurance) is commercially sold insurance that is specifically tailored to provide additional coverage to people on Medicare. These policies must meet certain minimum standards set by federal law and enforced by the states through their departments of insurance.

Medicare supplement policies cover some but not all of the gaps in Medicare. They typically pay for deductibles and co-payments. Some policies also pay for one or two services that are not covered by Medicare, such as care in foreign countries, prescription drugs, or eyeglasses. Medicare supplement policies do not, however, cover expenses for long-term care.

There are dozens of Medicare supplement policies on the market. They vary in what they will pay for, in how soon they will cover pre-existing conditions, in your right to renew the policy, and in how healthy or young you need to be to qualify for them.

Coverage

Medicare supplement policies are designed primarily to cover the deductibles and co-payments for which Medicare beneficiaries are responsible. For Part A services, nearly all Medicare supplement policies will cover the $592 hospital deductible, the 25 percent co-payment for days 61 to 90, and the 50 percent co-payment for the lifetime reserve days. Most will also cover at least 90 percent of the hospital expenses for 365 days after all Medicare hospital benefits are exhausted. Some policies will cover the $74 co-payment for days 21 to 100 in a skilled nursing facility and provide skilled nursing facility coverage after 100 days.

For Part B services, some Medigap policies will cover the $75 Part B deductible; others will not. Nearly all policies will pay the 20 percent co-payment on Medicare-approved charges. In addition, some policies will pay for a portion of excess charges. This may or may not be important, depending on whether you live in an area with an abundance of doctors who accept Medicare assignment.

Apart from one or two extra services (see p. 28), Medicare supplement policies will pay only for the services covered by Medicare. If Medicare won't pay for a service, the Medicare supplement policy is unlikely to pay either.

Pre-existing Conditions

If you have a serious medical condition that needs ongoing treatment or one that may need treatment at any time, be sure to pay special attention to how policies cover pre-existing conditions. A pre-existing condition is a medical condition that you have been treated for, or one that you knew existed, before the effective date of a policy.

Some policies will cover pre-existing conditions immediately. Others will make you wait one to six months before they will begin to pay for such conditions. Some insurance companies will allow you to buy riders that provide coverage immediately for pre-existing conditions.

Underwriting

Once you are on Medicare, it's relatively easy to buy supplemental insurance. Because Medicare will pay for such a large portion of your medical expenses if you are ill, most insurance companies are eager to sell additional medical insurance to the elderly—so eager that many companies don't require a physical exam or a doctor's statement before issuing coverage. Some companies even accept all applicants, with no questions asked.

Certain companies are more selective about who they will insure and accept only applicants who are relatively healthy or not much older than 65. This process is known as underwriting. A company that selects only healthy or younger applicants may charge lower rates. But keep in mind that unless the policy protects you from cancellation, the company might refuse to renew your policy when you no longer meet its strict criteria.

If you are turned down by one company, don't be discouraged. If you are reasonably healthy, you won't have a problem finding a company that will accept you. Only the very ill will find it difficult to secure coverage.

Renewability

Policies also differ in terms of whether the company can refuse to renew the policy. Some policies are "guaranteed renewable," meaning that the company cannot cancel your policy as long as you pay the premium. Other policies are "conditionally renewable," meaning the company is entitled to cancel the policy, but only if it also cancels all of the policies in the same class. For example, if a policy is conditionally renewable, the company cannot single you out for cancellation, but it can decide to cancel all of the policies sold in your state.

Some policies have no protection against cancellation. Obviously, guaranteed renewable policies are desirable because they offer the most protection against cancellation.

CHOOSING WHICH SUPPLEMENTAL INSURANCE IS BEST FOR YOU

If you decide to buy Medicare supplement insurance, you will find a large—and confusing—number of policies to choose from. Which one you buy should depend on your individual circumstances and how much risk you are able or willing to assume. (See Chapter 4.) Your decision should take into consideration your age, health, need for particular services, whether your doctors have agreed to accept Medicare assignment, how easy it is to find other doctors in your community who accept assignment, and how much you can afford to pay. Keep in mind that it is unwise and probably unaffordable to buy insurance that will close all of the gaps. Use the worksheet in Appendix C to help you identify the features that you need in a policy before you begin shopping. If you buy a policy, you should concentrate your dollars in one good policy. More policies do not mean more protection.

POLICIES TO AVOID

Some of the policies that insurance companies sell to senior citizens are not designed to supplement Medicare. Most of them are heavily advertised, and they include hospital indemnity policies, medical-surgical insurance, accident insurance, and cancer and other dread-disease policies. Playing on our natural anxieties about being unable to afford good health care in the event of serious illness, many of the companies try to convince seniors that these policies offer valuable protection, when in fact they are of nearly no help in covering serious expenses. Seniors should avoid these policies because the benefits they offer are extremely limited, and in many cases they fail to keep up with inflation. Their general provisions are described in what follows.

Hospital Indemnity Insurance

Hospital indemnity policies pay a set amount of money (usually $20 to $100) for each day you are hospitalized. Some indemnity policies provide even narrower coverage, paying only if you are confined to an intensive-care unit or need emergency treatment. These policies are relatively inexpensive, and for a good reason. They provide no real protection.

The benefits you receive from these policies (if any) are likely to be small. For seniors, the average hospital stay is about nine days. Stays of more than 20 days are extremely rare. The benefits these policies pay for each day are almost negligible compared to the average actual cost of hospitalization—over $900 per day.

Remember that most hospital bills are covered by Medicare. If you have large medical bills that do not involve hospitalization, hospital indemnity policies pay nothing. Moreover, since the amount these policies pay per day is fixed, the value of the policy is steadily eaten away by inflation. What starts out as a poor policy becomes even less valuable every year.

Medical-Surgical Insurance

Sometimes sold as a rider to hospital indemnity insurance, medical-surgical policies aimed at seniors pay for the same services as Medicare Medical Insurance (Part B). These medical-surgical policies typically pay a fixed amount for each medical service you receive. For example, a policy might pay $300 for surgery to repair a broken hip. Like hospital indemnity policies, medical-surgical insurance is not designed to keep up with inflation. In addition, these policies often pay only $3,000 to $5,000 in total benefits. For most seniors, they are a bad buy.

Accident Insurance

Accident insurance pays a fixed amount in the event of death, dismemberment, or catastrophic injury resulting from an accident. These policies pay if there is a plane crash, train wreck, or other sudden disaster, but they usually pay nothing if you have a serious illness.

Cancer and Other Dread-Disease Insurance

Dread-disease policies pay only if you need treatment for a particular severe disease such as cancer. Buying one of these policies is gambling that you will contract precisely that disease, for these policies provide no coverage if you require treatment for any other reason. *Nor are you covered if you have already been diagnosed or treated for the disease.*

Medicare and a good, comprehensive Medicare supplement policy will cover hospital and medical costs that are caused by accidents, cancer, or other disease. Instead of wasting your money on these policies, you are better off concentrating your premium dollars in one good supplement policy.

HEALTH MAINTENANCE ORGANIZATIONS

In many areas, joining a Health Maintenance Organization (HMO) is an attractive alternative to buying supplemental insurance. An HMO operates like a combination health-care provider and insurance company. It provides health care to its members and charges them a fixed amount per month.

Nearly 100 HMOs have signed contracts with the federal

government agreeing to provide services to seniors enrolled in Medicare. Under these agreements, the government pays the HMO a fixed amount for each senior they sign up. In exchange, the HMO must provide these seniors with all of the Medicare-covered services they need. They are allowed to provide other services as well. The HMO charges seniors a monthly premium to cover the cost of deductibles, co-payments, and services not covered by Medicare.

There are some clear advantages to joining an HMO. For a fixed monthly fee, HMOs usually provide all of the services that you need. To induce seniors to join, some HMOs have added needed services such as eyeglasses and prescription drugs for only a small additional fee. Generally, there are no deductibles or excess charges to worry about. Where co-payments exist, they are usually small. There are no claim forms to fill out. In addition, unlike insurance companies, HMOs cannot reject you or charge you more because of your age or health. HMOs sign up applicants during "open enrollment periods." During those periods, they are required to accept applicants on a first-come, first-served basis.

Joining an HMO has a few disadvantages. If you sign up, you are locked into the HMO for medical care. *You must use only the HMO for all covered services.* Medicare will not pay for covered services by any other provider. If you use any other doctors or hospitals, you are responsible for paying the entire bill. (Most HMOs will pay for emergency care if you are traveling outside of your particular service center's area.)

Another disadvantage is that if the HMO decides not to renew its Medicare contract, you may need to find new doctors and new insurance in a hurry. Twenty-four HMOs that had Medicare contracts in 1988 decided not to renew them in January 1989, affecting more than 58,000 Medicare enrollees. Most were smaller HMOs that were dissatisfied with the amount they were being paid per enrollee.

If you are interested in joining an HMO, your local Social Security office can give you the names of those with Medicare contracts in your area. You should contact the HMOs directly to find out what their services and fees are and when they will be accepting new members. Ask how long the HMO has been operating, when its Medicare contract expires, and how long it expects to continue to provide care to Medicare recipients. If you are told that an HMO's contract is about to expire in a few months and that it is unlikely to be renewed, look for another HMO.

Since you will have to receive all your care from the HMO, try to evaluate the HMO's service before you sign up. If you know anyone who belongs to it, ask about the service they are receiving. Some questions to ask are:

- How long do you have to wait when you need care?
- Are you assigned to a doctor who has overall responsibility for your care?
- Can you usually see that doctor when you make an appointment?
- Do the doctors available seem to take enough time to find out what's wrong, provide the right treatment, and answer your questions?
- Can you see a specialist when your condition requires one?
- Can you get through on the telephone to make an appointment?
- Is the staff helpful or indifferent when you need help?

Since people will be able to tell you only about their individual experiences with an HMO, talk to as many people as you can.

BEFORE YOU BUY

Before you buy a policy or sign up for an HMO, check whether you are already covered. Some employer group health plans cover employees and their spouses after retirement. Certain plans continue to provide full or nearly full coverage, while others automatically convert to a Medicare supplement policy when an employee becomes eligible for Medicare.

If you are covered, examine the benefits available through your employer plan before you decide to reject them. Employer plans are not subject to the same laws as individual Medigap policies. Therefore, it is important to study them closely. Some employer plans offer better coverage at lower cost than policies you can buy on your own. Others offer relatively poor protection. Generally, group plans cover all pre-existing conditions. If the coverage is less than you would like, ask whether you can increase it by paying an additional premium. If the coverage is still inadequate, consider refusing the employer plan and buying a better Medigap policy.

If your spouse is younger and not yet eligible for Medicare but is covered by your employer plan, you may need to stay with the plan even if it is expensive. Many people who are approaching 65 and therefore not yet eligible for Medicare benefits cannot find any insurance companies to cover them. Those who manage to find coverage often pay extremely high premiums. Once your spouse is receiving Medicare, it should be easy to find supplemental coverage at an affordable price.

If your income is low enough to be eligible for Medicaid, do not buy supplemental insurance. The Medicaid program already covers your hospital and medical expenses. In some states, it is illegal to sell Medicare supplement insurance to someone who is eligible for Medicaid.

The rules for qualifying for Medicaid vary from state to state. In general, your assets (excluding your home) must be less than $1,900 ($2,800 for a couple) and your income must be less than about $300 a month ($425 for a couple). The amounts may be higher or lower, depending on where you live.

If your assets and income are low but not low enough to meet these requirements, keep in mind that any substantial medical expenses you incur might well deplete your assets to an extent that you will be eligible for Medicaid. For example, if the assets of you and your spouse (excluding your home) are $8,000, and your combined monthly income is $600, any illness that depletes your assets by $5,200 and your monthly income by $175 will qualify you for Medicaid. With annual premiums running about $1,000 per person, it makes little sense to buy Medicare supplement insurance. (See Chapter 11.)

4

Buying a Medicare Supplement Policy

Most seniors regularly receive information aimed at selling them some form of health insurance. The information comes from three sources: agents, companies who directly write insurance without using an agent, and organizations selling group insurance to their members.

Agents contact seniors by mail, telephone, and personal visits. Some agents sell only the policies of one particular company; others are so-called independent agents, who offer to find you the best policy for your needs from the many companies they represent. Be aware, however, that buying from an independent agent is no guarantee of obtaining the best policy for your situation, since many agents select policies solely on the basis of which ones pay them the highest commissions.

Some insurance companies don't use agents. Instead, they advertise their policies through television, magazine, and newspaper ads and send you cards and letters by mail. Though such companies can reduce costs because agent commissions are eliminated, not all companies pass these savings on to customers.

The third source of insurance consists of organizations offering group policies, which can provide lower costs because agent commissions are eliminated and the organization can bargain on behalf of its members. Again, it is the terms of the policy rather than the name or reputation of the organization that count. These group policies are usually offered by mailed solicitations from alumni associations, professional, trade, or union associations, and organizations that serve seniors.

Before contacting anyone who sells insurance, get as much information as possible from an insurance counseling program, if there is one serving your area, or from your state insurance commissioner. (See Appendix B.) These two independent sources can provide you with pamphlets and buying guides and help you evaluate policies sold in your state. They can also warn you about any unfair practices occurring in your community.

Once you have identified your insurance needs and some policies that might meet them, call or write the agent, company, or group offering the policy and ask them to send you an outline of coverage. The outline of coverage will identify the expenses a policy will pay for and how much it will pay. Reviewing the outline will help you decide whether a policy actually meets your needs.

With the independent information and outline of coverage in hand, you will be better prepared to buy a Medicare supplement policy.

<u>GENERAL RULES</u>

Here are some general rules to keep in mind when shopping for a supplement policy:

1. Know what you want to buy, and don't buy anything else. Some insurance agents are not interested in selling you a policy that is suitable to your individual needs. They are interested only in selling you the policy that pays them the biggest commission. Be sure to identify what you want from a policy before you go shopping. Don't let an agent talk you out of what you decided is important.

2. Compare the policies and prices offered by several companies and agents. You are more likely to find a policy that meets your needs by shopping around. Be wary of insurance agents (including so-called independent agents) who push only one policy rather than presenting a range of choices.

3. Know who you're dealing with. If possible, ask friends and relatives for the names of agents who have been helpful and trustworthy in the past. When you contact a company or agent, get the person's name (first and last), address, telephone number, and the name of the company or companies he or she is representing. Write this information down and keep it where you can find it if you have any questions or problems.

4. Insist that the company representative or agent give you a copy of the outline of coverage for each policy you are considering. Study the outline *before you make a decision.* Both companies and agents are required by law to give you a written outline of coverage that summarizes the benefits, exclusions, limitations, renewability, premiums, and other conditions for the policy that you are buying. Many buyers receive this information too late in the sales process to make a proper decision. Some states do not require that the outline be delivered until the buyer actually submits an application.

5. If you decide to buy a policy, buy one good one. Many seniors are led to believe that buying several policies means buying more protection. In nearly all cases, buying more than one policy is a waste of money. For every policy you buy, you are paying for more sales commissions, more advertising, and more insurance company profits. Consumers are better off buying one comprehensive Medicare supplement policy and not spending more than they need for company expenses.

6. Be careful how you replace an existing policy. Some policies will not cover pre-existing conditions for one to six months. If you are thinking about canceling a policy and replacing it with a new one, make sure that there is a good reason for switching. Also, be sure that the new policy covers pre-existing conditions, so that there is no time during which you are not covered. These precautions are crucial if you have a medical condition that requires ongoing treatment, or one that may need treatment at any time.

7. Check on your right to renew a policy. A policy that is "guaranteed renewable" cannot be canceled by the company as long as you pay your premium. At the end of a policy term (for example, one year), the company must renew your policy on the same terms and conditions, although it usually may increase your premium. If a policy is "conditionally renewable," the company cannot single you out for cancellation; it can cancel your policy only if it cancels all other policies in its class. A class may be large or small, depending on how the company has defined it. For example, a company might define a class as all women between the ages of 70 and 75 who were sold a policy in the state of Texas. A "cancelable" policy may be canceled at any time. Generally, companies are required to give you written notice at least 30 days before doing so. Obviously, a policy that is guaranteed renewable will give you the most protection against cancellation.

8. Be skeptical of claims concerning nursing-home coverage. Medicare supplement policies do not cover long-term care in nursing homes. These policies will cover medically intense but relatively short-term care in a skilled nursing facility. However, most policies provide no coverage for custodial care, which helps people with bathing, eating, dressing, taking medications, and performing other daily activities. Persons providing custodial care need less training than those providing skilled nursing care. Most seniors who need long-term care need custodial, rather than skilled nursing care. (For more information about long-term care, see Chapter 10.)

HOW TO READ A POLICY

When you receive your policy, read it carefully. The policy is a written contract between you and the insurance company. It will specify the expenses that the company will pay for, the exclusions and limitations that apply, the procedure for filing claims for covered expenses, and the company's right to cancel the policy.

In recent years, insurance companies have been prodded to rewrite their policies in plain language. A few states have passed laws requiring understandable policy language. Though some companies have rewritten their policies in plain language, others continue to use obscure terms and incomprehensible sentences in their policies.

As you read your policy, make sure that the coverage and the premium stated specify exactly what you have agreed to. Also, make sure that the policy does not include any restrictions, exclusions, or limitations that you did not expect. If you have any questions or doubts about the policy, ask others to read it as well. If there is an insurance counseling program in your area, ask its staff for advice.

A typical policy is organized as follows:

1. *Declarations.* This section states the name and address of the policyholder, the policy number, and the type, term, premium, and effective date of the policy. While this information is not complicated, it should be checked carefully.

2. *Description of coverage and benefits.* This section identifies the services that the company will pay for and any deductibles, co-payments, and maximum amounts that may apply. The information is sometimes presented in the form of a chart.

3. *Exclusions and limitations.* This section lists the services and medical conditions that the company will *not* pay for. Examine it closely and look for any "riders" or "endorsements" that may be attached to the policy. These attachments may change the exclusions and limitations specified in the policy itself.

4. *Waiting period.* This section describes how long you have to wait before the company will pay for expenses for pre-existing conditions. It will also provide its definition of pre-existing condition, for example, "any condition, disease, or ailment for which you had received medical treatment or advice six months before the effective date of your policy."

5. *How to use your benefits.* This section describes how to file a claim under the policy. It states what forms to use, what information to provide, and where to mail the claim.

6. *Cancellation.* This section describes the conditions under which the company may cancel your policy. It also describes how you can cancel the policy if you no longer want the coverage. This section is sometimes entitled "Termination of Benefits" or "Renewability."

7. *Riders.* Riders are additional pieces of paper attached to the policy that contain additional policy terms. Be sure to read all attachments. Riders may expand your coverage by providing additional benefits, or they may limit coverage by excluding certain services or conditions. Riders are sometimes referred to as "endorsements."

HOW TO CANCEL A POLICY

If you don't want the insurance for any reason, you should act quickly to cancel it. After you receive a policy, most states give you 30 days to examine it and return it to the insurance company for a full refund. You do not have to provide a reason for returning it.

To cancel a policy during this 30-day period: (1) write a letter to the company, stating that you want the policy canceled; (2) enclose the policy with the letter; and (3) mail the letter and policy directly to the company by certified mail. (A sample letter is shown in Appendix C.) Keep a copy of the letter and the return receipt from the post office for your records. The receipt is your proof that the policy was returned to the company during the cancellation period.

If you bought the policy through an agent, don't rely on the agent to cancel it for you. Some agents have tried to prevent seniors from canceling after agreeing to do so, then failing to notify the company within the 30-day period. Send your cancellation letter directly to the insurance company yourself.

If the insurance company does not respond to your letter

within 45 days (or responds, but only makes a partial refund), write a letter to your state insurance commissioner asking for help. If possible, identify the particular policy you bought, the date you received it, and the date you returned it. Enclose a copy of the cancellation letter you sent to the company and any written response from the company. If you talked with someone from the company, give that person's name, the date when you spoke to him or her, and what was said. If you don't have all of this information, be as specific as you can. (A sample letter can be found in Appendix C.) Keep a copy of the letter for your records.

5

How to Protect Yourself from Abusive Insurance Practices

An insurance agent convinces a Florida couple in their 80s to drop their existing insurance and buy policies costing four times as much. The agent tells them that the new policies will pay for all expenses not covered by Medicare, including total nursing-home coverage. When one of them becomes ill with Alzheimer's disease, they learn for the first time that the policies won't pay for custodial nursing care.

In Illinois, agents sell 28 Medicare supplement policies to an 88-year-old widow, including four different policies from the same insurance company. After a lengthy investigation by the state's department of insurance, the companies and agents are forced to refund nearly $10,000 they had collected in premiums.

In Mankato, Minnesota, agents from an insurance agency sell 14 health and life policies to an 80-year-old woman. Her only source of income is a monthly Social Security check for $217. For a year, her entire income goes to paying premiums for unnecessary policies.

In San Jose, California, senior citizens receive a mailing from the California Association for Concerned Senior Citizens, warning them of cuts in Medicare and urging them to buy a recommended policy. In fact, no such organization exists. The mailing comes from an insurance agency that sells Medicare supplement insurance.

In the state of Washington, senior citizens receive mailings that appear to be official government notices of cuts in Medicare benefits. The notices urge them to buy supplemental insurance and ask them to return a card to receive more information. The next thing they know, there's a sales agent at their door. In fact, the mailings are from an insurance company and two firms that develop and sell sales leads to insurance agents.

In Arlington, Virginia, a 68-year-old widow interviews a dozen local insurance agents as part of a congressional investigation into Medigap sales abuses. Eleven recommend that she cancel her existing policy and buy a new one, even though it will mean a new waiting period for pre-existing conditions. Only one tells her the truth—that she is adequately insured and there is no Medicare supplement policy that offers comprehensive protection against nursing-home expenses.

In Wheaton, Maryland, a couple depletes their life savings and turns to Medicaid to pay for nursing-home care. Between them, they have been paying for five Medicare supplement policies. None of the agents bothered to tell them that the policies would not pay for most kinds of nursing-home care.

In every community in every state, there are examples of seniors who have been subjected to scare tactics, fraud, deception, and other abusive marketing practices by insurance companies and agents. These companies and agents often prey on seniors who fear that they won't have sufficient money to pay for essential hospital and medical expenses. A 1986 congressional report estimates that senior citizens lose $3 billion annually because of such abusive marketing practices. Seniors can help protect themselves by raising their awareness of these possible abuses and taking some preventive measures.

BUYING INSURANCE FROM AGENTS

While all insurance agents are not scoundrels, many who sell Medicare supplement policies to seniors are either incompetent or willing to use unfair and deceptive practices. Some try to bully or frighten elderly people into buying one or more policies. Others use friendly smiles and personal attention to gain a buyer's trust.

Buying insurance is a business transaction. If you are interested in buying insurance from an agent, schedule a meeting in the agent's office. If the agent offers to come to your home, decline the offer, if possible. You are more likely to be caught off guard in your home; agents are business people and should have an office. No matter where the meeting takes place, set a definite date for it and a definite time for it to begin and end. Stick to that schedule.

Bring a person you trust to the meeting. He or she does not have to be an insurance expert. Someone who can think clearly and is not afraid of jumping in when help is needed will do fine. The agent may try to confuse you. If so, two heads are better than one. Both of you should read this chapter before the meeting so that you know what to watch out for.

Be sure to interview several agents and ask each of them to give you the written outline of coverage for each policy they are recommending. When you have several outlines, sit down and go over the materials with a friend. When you have selected the policy that you want to buy, contact the agent selling that policy for an application.

Keep in mind that just because an agent has spent some time with you does not obligate you to buy from that agent. Buy from an agent only if you feel that he or she is both competent and trustworthy and that the policy he or she is selling is suitable for you. A responsible agent will encourage you to take your time in making important decisions and will not object when you want another opinion. If you have any doubts about an agent, find another one.

Danger Signs

When you are dealing with agents, watch out for the following danger signs. If you see any of these signs, take your business elsewhere at once. To prevent the agent from victimizing other seniors, file a complaint with your state insurance commissioner or contact law enforcement officials.

1. The agent says that he or she works for Medicare or some other government agency. For years, many insurance agents have tried to sell policies by suggesting that they either work for Medicare or are somehow associated with the Medicare program. Any such statement or suggestion is false and illegal. Refuse to do business with any agent who tries this ploy.

2. The agent tries to sell you a policy without asking what kind of insurance you have already, or without taking time to examine your existing insurance. The law prohibits an agent from knowingly selling you overlapping insurance coverage. One way some agents get around the law is by not asking about your current insurance. A conscientious agent will always carefully check your existing coverage before making any recommendations.

3. The agent says that his or her policy will cover 100 percent of the expenses not covered by Medicare. The agent is either lying or has not done enough homework to help you. Even the most comprehensive policy will cover only some of the gaps left by Medicare. No policy will provide you with 100 percent Medigap coverage. Agents who encourage you to plug every gap with some kind of insurance will waste a lot of your money. Remember that it is impractical (and unaffordable) to close all the gaps in Medicare; your goal should be to close only the most important ones, given your individual situation. Achieving that goal requires thought, planning, and an accurate knowledge of the policies on the market.

4. The agent asks that you pay in cash. Some agents have pocketed seniors' money without securing any coverage. Always pay your insurance premiums by check. Premium checks should be made out to the insurance company, not the agent.

5. The agents asks you for a personal loan. Some financially strapped agents have taken advantage of their close relationship with a client by asking for a personal loan. Unless you are willing to lose your money, don't make loans to agents, even for a short amount of time.

6. The agent refuses to leave his or her business card, brochure, or outline of coverage. Some agents try to cover their tracks by refusing to leave any materials with the buyer. Many agents who engage in abusive sales practices will not leave their business cards or any misleading sales literature they may have shown you so that it is more difficult for buyers to file complaints. Some agents also refuse to leave truthful materials in case they might disclose that you are getting less than what you believe you're buying.

7. The agent tries to scare or bully you into buying a policy. If you feel that an agent is trying to scare, pressure, or intimidate you into buying a policy, leave immediately or end the interview if the agent is in your home. If the agent attempts to keep you from leaving or does not leave as quickly as you would like, threaten to call the police. If the agent offers to drive you to the bank to get or transfer funds, refuse the offer. If you did agree to buy a policy simply to get rid of a bullying agent, notify the bank to stop payment on the check and write the insurance company to cancel the policy. These situations may seem extreme, but many seniors have had to deal with agents who use tactics like these to make a sale.

8. The agent attempts to sell you more than one policy, or to replace an existing policy, when there is no good reason to do

so. If the agent tells you that there is a reason, insist that he or she put it in writing so that you can discuss it with others. Be skeptical, and don't be rushed into buying.

9. An agent shows up at your door unsolicited to sell you insurance. Some agents actively look for seniors who may be interested in buying more insurance. One way for them to identify these seniors is to get them to return a card requesting more information about Medicare.

The highly competitive search for insurance buyers has given rise to companies that specialize in mailing deceptive notices to senior citizens. Some of these mailings are designed to look like official government notices informing seniors of drastic cuts in Medicare. The mailings urge seniors to return a card with their name and address to receive more information about how they can protect themselves against costly medical expenses.

If you respond to one of these mailings by sending in a card, your card will be sold to an insurance agent. The agent who buys your card may call you and tell you that he or she is responding to your request for information and then ask to come and see you. Or the agent may just knock on your door without calling you first.

Some agents will contact you without telling you that they got your name from a card that you mailed months ago. They may say that they are from your present insurance company, or tell you that your own agent has died and they are coming to review the coverage, even though these are lies. Their goal, of course, is to sell you more insurance.

Be skeptical about unsolicited sales calls. Reputable agents with well-established businesses usually call on people only when their services have been requested.

Many people feel embarrassed when they discover that they have been tricked by an unscrupulous agent. Often, they blame themselves for not being smarter, quicker, or more perceptive. But even a knowledgeable person can be deceived at times by an agent who is willing to lie, steal, or exploit one's trust.

If you think that an agent has engaged in any unfair or deceptive practice, stop that agent from victimizing others. Get help. State insurance regulators have the power to revoke or suspend an agent's license. They also can order refunds and seek fines. District attorneys and attorneys general have the authority to bring criminal charges against agents or seek civil injunctions and monetary penalties. If law enforcement officials won't act or the existing local laws are too weak, your legislator can push for stronger enforcement or introduce tougher measures to deal with abusive agents. (Appendix B describes these and other resources that may be helpful.)

You should also consider talking to a local reporter about the problems you have had. A news story could help to warn other seniors in your community and focus public attention on the need to prevent agents from engaging in the types of activities described in this chapter.

BUYING INSURANCE BY MAIL

Some insurance companies sell policies directly to seniors, bypassing the agents. These companies promote their policies through newspaper and magazine advertisements, television ads, and direct mail to seniors. Potential buyers receive information by mail, complete an application, mail it to the company with a premium, and receive their policy in the mail.

Buying insurance by mail has several possible advantages. By eliminating agents' commissions, the insurance company has lower costs and may pass some of this savings on to you in the form of lower premiums or better coverage. In addition, by eliminating commissioned sales agents, companies may avoid the abuses associated with some agents.

However, insurance companies have not always lived up to this potential. While some policies sold by mail offer good protection and value, others are mediocre or worse. Even though there are no abusive agents to contend with, some insurance companies have engaged in marketing abuses of their own. At times, advertising by these companies has been either misleading or purposely designed to frighten seniors into buying policies.

If you are considering buying an insurance policy by mail, request a copy of the outline of coverage and examine it closely. Don't decide to buy on the basis of advertisements alone, or because the policy is endorsed by a celebrity. Insurance companies that use celebrity endorsements are attempting to get people to buy on the basis of emotion and blind trust, rather than a hard look at what they are selling. Just because someone hosted a television show does not mean that he or she cares—or even knows—whether you get a good policy. Like insurance agents, celebrities are paid to sell products, whether dog food or insurance policies.

Be skeptical of ads that say "Limited Offer!" or "Offer Expires in 30 Days!" or "Last Chance!" Companies periodically run these ads to pressure people to buy. Remember, even if a particular policy is discontinued, there are many policies on the market. Don't be rushed.

If you decide to buy, pay by check. If the policy you receive is not what you thought you were getting, or if you change your mind about buying it, use your 30-day right to cancel the policy.

BUYING INSURANCE THROUGH A GROUP

Some supplemental policies are available through a group or an organization. But buying a policy through a group does not automatically guarantee that you are buying a good policy. Often, the term "group" is simply a marketing device.

Hospital indemnity policies, for example, are often sold as "group insurance" to people who have nothing in common except that they are holders of department store credit cards. A common inducement is to offer the first month of coverage for only a dollar. At any price, hospital indemnity policies are a waste of money, and buying a hospital indemnity policy through a group doesn't make it any better.

Even sponsorship by a well-known organization is no guarantee that you are buying the best policy for your particular needs. Over the years, the American Association of Retired Persons (AARP) has sold a number of different policies that have varied in quality.

If you are considering buying a policy through a group, ask about renewability. Most of these policies are only "conditionally renewable," meaning that the insurance company writing the policy could cancel the whole group. If that happened, the group may be able to find new coverage from another company, but the terms and premiums offered may be different. The new policy might not suit your individual needs. Staying aware of your own particular situation is sometimes difficult when you are being showered by the flattering attentions of group identification. But sometimes it's necessary if you're to find the insurance that's right for you.

6

When You Get a Bill

After eight days in the hospital, followed by more than three weeks in a nursing home, Mrs. A went home. The hip she had broken still hurt, although less each day. She could now stand for a short time, but normal walking was impossible. Months of rehabilitation were still ahead of her.

At home, Mrs. A found a stack of bills. There were bills from three doctors: her family doctor, who saw her a number of times after her accident; the surgeon who operated on her hip; and a third doctor, whose name was unfamiliar to her. There were also bills from the hospital, the nursing home, a physical therapist, the ambulance service, and the medical equipment company.

Mixed in with the bills were some envelopes from Medicare, all of which contained Explanations of Medical Benefits (EOMBs). Some also contained checks made out to her. Mrs. A read all of the EOMBs, but she still wasn't sure which bills Medicare had paid and which ones were still outstanding. She decided to deposit the checks right away so she wouldn't lose them and began to work on the papers a little each day.

Even an illness less severe than Mrs. A's can produce a pile of bills. In addition to the bill from your doctor, there may be bills from a hospital, a clinic, one or more specialists, an anesthesiologist, a clinical lab, a rehabilitation therapist, a home health agency, an equipment supplier, and an ambulance service.

Some of these bills may have been sent to Medicare for direct payment; if so, you do not need to do anything about them. Other bills may be due when you receive them, or soon after. For still other bills, you may need to submit a claim to Medicare or to your Medigap insurer. (Chapter 7 explains how to submit a claim.) The key to dealing with your bills is knowing which ones you need to pay right away, which ones have already been paid, and which ones should not be paid until a later date.

ORGANIZING YOUR BILLS

The first step is to sort the bills into two stacks. Bills for services covered by Part A (inpatient hospital care, inpatient skilled nursing-facility care, hospice care, and home health care) should be put in one stack. Bills for services covered by Part B (doctors' services, outpatient hospital services, lab tests, durable medical equipment, ambulance service, etc.) go in another stack.

Next, sort your bills according to which facility provided the service being charged. Take the bills covered by Part A and make a separate stack for each of these providers. Put hospital bills in one stack, the skilled nursing-home bills in another, and so on. If you have more than one bill from the same provider, sort them by the date they were sent, with the oldest bill on the bottom and the most recent bill on top. Put a clip or rubber band around each provider stack. Do the same with the bills for services covered by Part B. Make separate stacks for each doctor, clinic, lab, and so on, with the oldest bill on the bottom and the most recent ones on top.

If you received any papers from Medicare, sort these as well. Separate them into two piles: one for Part A services (inpatient hospital and skilled nursing-home services) and one for Part B services (doctors' services, lab services, etc.). You should be able to do this easily, since the forms look quite different. Put each stack in chronological order, with the oldest papers on the bottom and the most recent ones on top.

You now have the foundation for an organized system for dealing with your bills. The next step is to determine which bills have already been paid, which need to be paid right away, and which should not be paid until a later date.

PAYING PART-A BILLS
(HOSPITAL, SKILLED NURSING HOME,
HOSPICE, AND HOME HEALTH CARE)

For services covered by Part A, the hospital, skilled nursing home, hospice, or home health agency will send the bill directly to Medicare. Medicare will then pay the provider 100 percent of the Medicare-approved charge for the service, less anything you owe for a deductible, a co-payment, or for services not covered. For most services, you will receive a Medicare Benefit Notice stating how much Medicare paid. The notice will also tell you how much you owe for any deductibles, co-payments, and services not covered. The provider will send you a bill for your portion. *This* is the amount you are responsible for. Remember that home health agencies receive all of their reimbursement from Medicare. They cannot bill you for additional amounts.

When many hospitals bill Medicare, they will also send you an itemized bill. Some hospitals will stamp these bills with a notice stating that Medicare has been billed and that they do not expect payment of the portion you owe until after Medicare has paid its portion. In this case, don't attempt to pay the hospital based on the itemized bill. Instead, wait until Medicare has paid its share. You will receive a Medicare Benefit Notice followed by a new bill from the hospital that reflects the Medicare payment. Pay only the amount of the new bill. If you were in the hospital for less than 60 days, you should not have to pay more than $592 (in 1990) in hospital expenses. If you are asked to pay more than this amount, call the hospital and ask them to explain the reason.

PAYING PART-B BILLS (DOCTORS' SERVICES,
LAB TESTS, MEDICAL EQUIPMENT, ETC.)

Bills for services covered by Part B are handled in one of two ways. If the doctor, clinic, equipment company, or other provider has agreed to accept Medicare assignment, the process is similar to that used to pay Part-A bills. If the provider has not agreed to accept assignment, the provider will submit a claim to Medicare for you. Medicare will send you a check for its share of the covered services and you are responsible for paying the bill.

Bills for Assigned Services

If the provider agrees to accept Medicare assignment, it will bill Medicare directly for the services. Medicare will pay the provider an amount based on an approved charge less any deductible or co-payment that you owe. Medicare then will send you an Explanation of Medical Benefits that states the amount it paid the provider; the applicable deductible and co-payments for which you are responsible; claims, if any, that it denied; and the reason for denying them.

After the provider has been paid by Medicare, you will be billed for the portion you owe. In most instances, this should be limited to any deductible or co-payment due. Providers who have agreed to accept Medicare assignment are not allowed to bill you for excess charges or to charge you fees for submitting claims to Medicare. If Medicare denies a claim because it decides that the services were unnecessary, you are not required to pay the bill for those services.

Charges for clinical lab services, whether provided by an independent lab or a doctor's office, must not exceed the amounts approved by Medicare, and bills must be sent by the provider directly to Medicare for payment. By law, you are not responsible for paying these charges.

Bills for Unassigned Services

After September 1, 1990, if a provider does not accept assignment, it will submit a claim to Medicare for you and also will send you a bill for its services. In most cases, you are responsible for paying the provider the entire billed amount, including any excess charges. Medicare will send you a reimbursement for its approved charge for the services, less any deductible or co-payment due from you.

There are two important exceptions to this rule. If Medicare denies your claim because it decides that a doctor's services were unnecessary, you are not required to pay the bill for those services unless the doctor warned you in writing that Medicare will not pay. Also, doctors are required to give you a written notice prior to performing any elective surgery over $500. (Elective surgery is any surgery that can be scheduled in advance, is not an emergency, and if delayed, would not result in death or permanent impairment of health.) The notice must state the estimated charges for surgery, how much Medicare is expected to pay, and the amount you will have to pay. If your doctor doesn't give you this information, he or she cannot charge you more than the amount paid by Medicare. In both cases, if you already paid the doctor, you are entitled to a refund.

If you received unassigned services prior to September 1, 1990, you will need to submit a claim to receive reimbursement. Follow the steps outlined in Chapter 7 for filing a Medicare form.

BILLS YOU ARE UNCERTAIN ABOUT

If you received services from several providers, it may not be easy to identify them all from the bills you receive. You may not even have seen all of them face-to-face. For example, your doctor may have asked a specialist to examine a specimen or to read an X ray. You may have seen some providers only once. Similarly, if you were in the hospital, your doctor may have asked another doctor to examine you for a particular condition, or an associate of your regular doctor may have visited you on a day when he or she was not available. Because it may be difficult to remember such providers, you may be surprised when you receive a bill for their services.

If you do receive a bill that you are not certain about, call the provider and ask what the bill is for. Also ask the provider whether he or she will bill Medicare directly or whether you are expected to submit the claim. For services covered by Part B (most notably, doctors' services), be sure to ask whether the provider will accept Medicare assignment, particularly if you have a lot of bills or large expenses.

KEEPING TRACK OF YOUR BILLS

Even if you have only a few bills, it helps to have a system to keep track of them. We recommend that you use the form in Appendix C to record and organize the information on your bills. Using this tracking form will enable you to determine whether you have been billed correctly and whether the correct amount has been paid by Medicare and any other insurance you have. (See Chapter 13 for suggestions about an easy general filing system.)

DEALING WITH OVERDUE BILLS

As time passes, you may receive notices that your account is past due, then letters demanding payment, and even a telephone call from the provider's bookkeeper or billing department, asking you to clear your account. These requests for payment can be intimidating.

If you need more time, call or write the provider and explain the situation. ("Your $15,000 bill for surgery is more than I can pay out of my own pocket. But several weeks ago, I submitted claims to both Medicare and my supplemental insurance. I will pay you as soon as I receive their checks. In the meantime, I'd appreciate it if you would stop the letters demanding immediate payment. Thanks for your assistance.") Most providers will be reasonable and give you the time you need.

If more time won't solve the problem, you may need to negotiate with the provider to accept a smaller fee, or to agree to payment in small installments. If the collection effort is too aggressive, you may need help from others. (See Chapter 9.) In any case, try not to feel anxious when confronted with sometimes intimidating billing procedures; usually a workable solution can be found to settle such demands.

7

How to File a Claim

Even if you are covered by Medicare and have supplemental insurance, neither will do you much good if you can't get the benefits you are entitled to. Knowing when and what to do if your claim is lost or denied is essential to obtaining these benefits.

WHEN TO FILE A MEDICARE CLAIM

The only time you need to file a claim with Medicare is if you received Part-B services from doctors and other providers who did not accept Medicare assignment prior to September 1, 1990. After September 1, 1990, claims will be submitted to Medicare for you by the health-care provider. You do not have to file a claim with Medicare. For services covered by Part A (inpatient hospital care, skilled nursing-home care, home health services, and hospice care) and for services covered by Part B that are provided under assignment, the provider will bill Medicare for you, and Medicare will pay the provider directly. For unassigned Part-B services (for example, unassigned doctors' services), the provider will submit a claim to Medicare for you. Medicare will send you a check for its share of the covered services and you are responsible for paying the provider.

COMPLETING THE MEDICARE CLAIM FORM

If you need to submit a claim for services you received before September 1, 1990, complete a Patient's Request for Medical Payment (Form 1490S). Copies are available either from the facility that provided the service or from your local Social Security office. Be sure to fill in your name and Medicare identification number *exactly* as they appear on your Medicare card. Sign and date the form. (See Appendix C.)

Next, attach your itemized bill(s) to the claim form. You can make a claim either before or after you pay the bills. Indicate which bills you have paid. You can attach *any* number of bills to the Patient's Request for Medical Payment. The bills do *not* have to be related; they can be from different providers and even for different illnesses. Each bill you attach must show the following information:

1. the name and address of the person or facility that provided the service

2. a description of the services you received and a procedure code for those services. The procedure code is important because it identifies the precise service you received. (For example, the code for a common office visit is 90050, and for a comprehensive office visit, 90060.)

3. the date you received the services

4. the place you received the services (for example, doctor's office, hospital, skilled nursing home, outpatient clinic, your home, etc.)

5. the amount charged for each service

6. your name and Medicare identification number

If you are making a claim for the purchase or rental of durable medical equipment, you must include your doctor's prescription and the itemized bill from the supplier. The prescription must describe the equipment you are buying or renting, give the medical reason for the equipment, and estimate how long you will need the equipment.

If any of this information is missing, your claim could be rejected or delayed, or Medicare could pay you a smaller amount than you are entitled to. For example, when a procedure code is missing, Medicare will often assign a code that results in the lowest payment, leaving you to pay the difference.

Most providers are familiar with Medicare claims requirements and will include this information automatically in all of their bills. Nevertheless, it's a good idea to check your bills. If any of the required information is missing, call the provider's office and ask for a bill that you can submit to Medicare.

Some providers will give you an itemized bill each time you receive services and also send you a monthly statement of the balance owed. Generally, Medicare will not pay on the basis of a statement that simply states a "balance forward." If you don't have an itemized bill, be sure to call the provider's office and ask for one.

WHERE TO SEND THE CLAIM

When you file a claim with Medicare, you are actually sending it to a large insurance company. For example, if you live in Illinois, you will send your Medicare claims to Blue Cross and Blue Shield of Illinois. The Medicare program hires companies like Blue Cross, Blue Shield, Aetna, and Prudential to review and pay Medicare claims. Companies that handle Hospital Insurance (Part A) claims are known as *intermediaries*, and companies that handle Medical Insurance (Part B) claims are known as *carriers*.

Because most of your claims will be for doctors' services, you will be dealing mostly with a Medical Insurance carrier. When you sign up for Medicare, a carrier will be assigned to you based on where you live. (For a complete list of carriers, see Appendix A.) Mail your claim to the Medical Insurance carrier for your area, and be sure to include the word *Medicare* in the carrier's address. If the claim is for a large amount, use registered mail so that you can have proof that it was delivered. Before sending off your claim, make a copy of the claim form and of all the attachments. Be sure to note the date you mail the claim, so you can follow up if there is no response.

Probably the only time you will need to deal with an intermediary (those who handle Part-A claims) is if you have a question about a Hospital Insurance claim or want to appeal one. (See Chapter 8.)

TIME LIMIT FOR SUBMITTING CLAIMS

You have at least 15 months from the time you receive medical care to submit a claim for it to Medicare. Use the table below to calculate how long you have to send in a claim.

DEADLINE FOR FILING MEDICARE CLAIMS

For services you receive between	Your claim must be submitted by
October 1, 1988, and September 30, 1989	December 31, 1990
October 1, 1989, and August 1, 1990	December 31, 1991

For services received after September 1, 1990, the provider is required to submit the claim for you.

Even though the rules give you lots of time, it's a good idea to get your claim in as soon as you can. It is much easier to file a claim when the services you've used are still fresh in your mind. In addition, as months go by, you may lose or misplace some of the bills.

HOW LONG WILL MEDICARE TAKE TO PAY MY CLAIM?

It generally takes Medicare carriers two to four weeks to process a claim. Some claims take longer. By law, Medicare carriers are required to pay 95 percent of those claims without any defect within 24 days.

When the carrier receives your claim, it will determine which services are covered by Medicare, compute the Medicare-approved charge, and calculate the amount owed you (taking into account any deductibles and co-payments for which you are responsible). The carrier will then send you a check and an Explanation of Medical Benefits (EOMB). The EOMB will show

- the name of the provider
- the date the services were provided
- the amount billed
- the amount approved for payment
- services that were paid
- services that were disallowed and the reasons for the disallowance
- any deductibles or co-payments that applied, and
- any deductible amount left after processing that claim

The provider's name on the EOMB can be a source of some confusion. For example, assume your doctor, Dr. Green, practices with Dr. Brown. Even though you see Dr. Green, Dr. Brown's name might appear on the EOMB simply because hers is the first name in the practice. (See Appendix C.)

In most cases, the check will be for 80 percent of the Medicare-approved charge for covered services, less any part of the $75 deductible you have not met. You are responsible for the deductible, the remaining 20 percent of the approved charge, and any amount over the approved charge. (For more information about the Part-B deductible and co-payments, see pages 23–24. If you have a Medicare supplement policy or other supplemental insurance, you may need to submit a claim to the insurance company.

If you don't hear from the carrier within 30 days of when your claim was mailed, call the carrier and ask for the reason for the delay. All Medicare carriers are required to have toll-free numbers to handle inquiries from the people they serve. (See Appendix A.)

WHAT IF MEDICARE DENIES MY CLAIM?

About one in every five claims processed by Medicare carriers is denied in whole or in part. For example, a carrier might deny a claim if it decided that the services were not covered by Medicare. Or it might pay a reduced amount if it felt that the services provided were excessive.

Even though EOMBs are supposed to explain why a claim is denied, the reasons provided in these notices are not always clear. If after reading the EOMB you are not sure why your claim was denied, call the carrier and ask for a further explanation. (The toll-free telephone number is usually at the top of the notice.) Be sure to have the EOMB and a copy of your claim in front of you when you call. Tell the company's representative that you would like to know exactly why your claim was denied.

If your claim is simple, the person who is helping you may be able to tell you the reason right away. If there is a problem, you may even be told on the telephone how to correct it so that your claim can be paid. If your claim is complicated or unusual, the representative may need several days to do some research and call you back.

If, after you receive an answer from the carrier, you still believe that you are entitled to payment, you have the right to appeal the carrier's decision. Unfortunately, mistakes are common, and sometimes the only way to correct them is to appeal. (For more information on how to appeal, see Chapter 8.)

Some problems are simple ones that usually can be corrected without an appeal. For example, many claims are denied because claimants forgot to sign their claim form, wrote down the wrong Medicare identification number, or made some other common mistake when preparing their claim. If your claim was denied because of an error like this, simply correct the mistake and send in the claim again. The carrier will usually pay the corrected claim.

If there is some question about the particular services you received, ask the doctor's staff at the facility that provided the service to help you figure out why the claim has been denied. For example, sometimes an insurance carrier will think that a claim duplicates another billing when, in fact, you received the same or similar services on more than one occasion. Getting the provider involved is often the only way to correct that kind of problem. Also, be aware that if your claim is denied because the services were considered unreasonable or unnecessary, you may not have to pay the provider. (For more information on bills that you don't have to pay, see Chapter 9.)

WHAT IF MY CLAIM IS LOST?

If you call the insurance carrier after 30 days and the representative says your claim was never received, you will have to start again. Ask your provider to submit another claim to Medicare.

For services received before September 1, 1990, you will have to fill out another Patient's Request for Medical Payment. Make new copies of the itemized bills you copied earlier and attach them to your request. Medicare guidelines require carriers to accept photocopies of itemized bills as long as there is no evidence of alteration.

Write a short note to the carrier explaining that the originals were lost in the mail. Double-check the carrier's address, then mail the claim to the carrier. If the claim is for a large amount, this time send it by registered mail. Be sure you note the date you mail the second claim, so you can follow up if there's no response in 30 days.

WHAT IF MEDICARE LATER
DECIDES IT PAID TOO MUCH?

On rare occasions, the insurance carrier might decide that it paid you too much. If such a mistake is discovered, then the carrier may send you a letter asking that you return the overpayment. If that attempt fails, the government may try to collect the overpayment by deducting it from your future Medicare benefits or from your Social Security retirement check.

If you believe that there was no overpayment, you can appeal the decision. (See Chapter 8.) Carriers have been instructed not to try to recover overpayments that are either too small (less than $10) or too old (paid more than four years ago). Moreover, the government won't insist on repayment if you can show that (1) you weren't at fault, and (2) you need the money for ordinary living expenses, or requiring you to pay would be unfair.

Since, in most cases, the carrier was entirely to blame for the overpayment, it is not too difficult for the Medicare beneficiary to show unfairness. For example, assume that a carrier states that you were overpaid $500 and tries to collect that amount from you three years later. If repayment would be a financial hardship, you should write to the carrier and ask that repayment be waived. Point out that the overpayment was not your fault and, if you can, include specific information about what the funds were used for and why you cannot afford to repay the amount they are trying to collect. Depending on the situation, the carrier may respond by waiving collection entirely, or by agreeing to collect the amount in small monthly installments over a number of years.

HOW OTHER BILLS ARE HANDLED

For services covered by Part A (inpatient hospital, skilled nursing, home health, and hospice care) and assigned services covered by Part B, the provider will bill the intermediary or the carrier for you. When the intermediary or the carrier receives the claim, it will compute the amount of payment due the provider (taking into account any deductibles and co-payments you are responsible for) and pay that amount to the provider directly. To let you know what it has paid, the intermediary or carrier will send you either a Medicare Benefit Notice (for inpatient hospital and skilled nursing-home services) or an Explanation of Medical Benefits (for other services).

After the provider has been paid by the intermediary, the provider will bill you for your portion. For example, if you are hospitalized for less than 60 days, your portion usually will be the

$592 hospital deductible. You are responsible for paying that portion to the provider. If you have a Medicare supplement policy or other supplemental insurance that covers the services provided, you may need to send a claim to the insurance company for all or part of your portion of the bill.

Occasionally, a provider may decide that the services are not covered by Medicare and may not submit a claim. For example, a nursing home might refuse to submit a claim to the intermediary because it has decided that the care you are receiving does not qualify as skilled nursing care.

If that happens, request that the provider submit a claim anyway so that the carrier or intermediary can make its own determination. If it denies the claim, you can appeal the decision. (For information on how to appeal, see Chapter 8.) *Make sure that the provider follows through and submits the claim. If the provider doesn't submit the claim, you will have no right to appeal.*

HOW TO SUBMIT A MEDICARE CLAIM FOR SOMEONE WHO HAS DIED

If a person who is covered by Medicare receives medical services but dies before submitting a claim, Medicare will still pay its share of covered services. Generally, the same rules apply. For services provided by a hospital, skilled nursing facility, home health agency, hospice, or other provider that accepts Medicare assignment, the provider will still bill Medicare directly and Medicare will pay its share to the provider. The provider will then bill the surviving spouse for any deductibles or co-payments. If there is no spouse, the provider will bill the patient's estate.

For other services (such as unassigned doctors' services), a spouse, son or daughter, other family member, or legal representative of the patient's estate may need to submit a claim on behalf of the deceased patient. To file a claim, you must fill out a Request for Information—Medicare Payment for Services to a Patient Now Deceased (Form HCFA 1660). That form will ask for information about whether the bills have been paid and who is responsible for unpaid bills. You must also complete a Patient's Request for Medical Payment (see Appendix C) and attach the bills for which you are seeking payment. These papers often get separated when they are being processed, so it's a good idea to write in large letters "HCFA 1660 ATTACHED" at the top of the claim and on each bill you send in. Mail the papers to the patient's carrier.

After September 1, 1990, providers are required to submit claims to Medicare for all covered services. This should eliminate the need to submit the Patient's Request for Medical Payment.

If the bills have been paid, the carrier will reimburse the person who paid the bills. If the patient paid the bills before he or she died, the carrier will pay the legal representative of the patient's estate, or if there is no representative, a surviving member of the patient's immediate family. For unpaid bills, the carrier will pay the person who has the legal obligation to pay, or whoever agrees to assume this obligation.

If there is no surviving spouse, or no estate to pay an outstanding bill, some providers will contact other family members and sometimes even friends and neighbors of the patient and attempt to make them feel morally responsible to pay. If you find yourself in that situation, don't give in. In most cases, you are not legally obligated to pay such bills. Remember that providers can always receive prompt payment directly from the Medicare carrier simply by submitting their bills as assigned claims. Of course, this would mean that they would have to forgo any charges that are in excess of the Medicare-approved amount.

YOUR RIGHT TO DISPUTE A BILL

A number of Medicare forms imply that you are obligated to pay a certain amount to the provider. For example, EOMBs will state an amount "owed Provider." HCFA Form 1600 states that the signer "assumes legal liability" for unpaid bills.

Remember, regardless of what these forms imply, you always have the right to dispute a bill that you believe is unfair. For example, if a provider bills you for an office visit, test, or other service that you did not receive, you have the right to refuse to pay the bill. The same is true if a provider promises to charge you a certain amount and then bills you for more. If the provider insists on payment, get some legal assistance. (See Appendix B.)

HOW TO SUBMIT A CLAIM
ON YOUR MEDICARE SUPPLEMENT POLICY

If you have a Medicare supplement policy, you will usually need to submit a claim to the insurance company after Medicare has paid its share. Most companies will require you to fill out a claim form. If you don't have forms, call the company and ask them to send you some.

Completing a claim form is usually a straightforward process, but it is important that the items be filled in correctly. Be sure to double-check any policy number, account number, or any other identifying number to make sure that it is correct.

Companies will usually require that you include copies of the Medicare Benefit Notices and EOMBs you have received. Some companies will also ask for copies of itemized bills. If itemized bills are requested, do not send statements that simply show a "balance due." In most cases, insurance companies will not pay claims based on these statements. Make a copy of your claim before you mail it to the company. Note the date you mail the claim.

Since Medicare has already examined your first set of claims and reported the results in the Medicare Benefit Notices or EOMBs, the insurance company should have an easy time processing claims on your supplemental insurance. If you don't receive a check within 30 days after you mailed the claim, call the company. If you don't receive a satisfactory answer about your claim, complain to your state insurance commissioner and the Health Care Financing Administration. (A sample letter is in Appendix C.)

Some companies now provide automatic claims handling, a process by which Medicare sends your Benefit Notices and

EOMBs directly to the insurance company. Payments should be even faster under this process, since it eliminates your having to receive these documents and send them on to the company. To find out whether your company has this service or is planning to offer it in the future, call the company.

WHEN TO BILL MEDICARE SECOND

If you are over 65, *still working,* and covered by your employer's group health plan, you must submit a claim to the employer plan *before* you file a claim with Medicare. (You can get claim forms from your employer.) After the employer plan has paid for the services that it covers, file a claim with your Medicare carrier. The carrier will pay for any Medicare-covered services that remain unpaid.

If you are still working and covered by an employer group plan, inform your doctor, hospital, and other providers so they will bill the plan first. If you are retired and covered by an employer plan, follow the normal rules and submit your claim to Medicare first.

These rules also apply to spouses covered by an employer group health plan. If you are married to someone who is *still working,* and you are covered by the employer's health plan, submit your claims to the employer plan first. If your spouse is retired, submit your claim to Medicare first.

If you are seeking Medicare benefits for treatment of a work-related illness or injury, or if you are covered by the Federal Black Lung Program for workers in the coal industry, you may also need to bill Medicare second. If you think you fit one of these descriptions, contract your carrier for instructions on how to proceed.

KEEPING UP WITH THE PAPERWORK

Filing claims can require a fair amount of paperwork. Forms need to be filled out. Copies of bills need to be sent and filed. Occasionally, you may need to write a letter to ask for an explanation or to straighten out something. None of this is fun, but it's the only way to get the benefits you are entitled to.

One way to make it easier is not to let the paperwork pile up. Handling just one or two pieces of paper at a time is manageable; facing a ten-inch stack is discouraging. It also helps to have a good filing system where you can put documents away and easily find them again. (See Chapter 13.)

8

Exercising Your Right
to Appeal

If your Medicare claim is denied by an insurance carrier or intermediary, you have the right to appeal. Over half of Medicare appeals result in either partial or total victory for the person appealing.

Although you can handle your own appeal, your chances of winning will be greatly improved if you contact a senior legal services program. (See Appendix B.) Many lawyers in these programs are familiar with the appeal process, and some are experts in the intricacies of the Medicare program. They can provide you with valuable advice and may even be willing to represent you. Contacting these programs also increases awareness of the kinds of problems seniors are having and may lead to a lawsuit, legislation, or other efforts to address the problem.

HOW TO APPEAL A PART-A CLAIM

If a hospital, skilled nursing home, home health-care agency, or hospice program files a claim on your behalf and the intermediary denies all or part of that claim, you have up to four opportunities to change that decision. Except for the last step, you can take all of these actions without the help of a lawyer.

Step 1: Reconsideration

If you disagree with the intermediary's decision, the first step is to make a "request for reconsideration." You must make the request *in writing* within 60 days after you receive notice of the intermediary's decision. You can request reconsideration regardless of how much money is involved in your claim.

To make the request, complete a Request for Reconsideration of Part A Hospital Insurance Benefits (Form HCFA 2649). (All of the forms referred to in this chapter are available from your local Social Security office. If you can't find the right form, write a brief letter saying that you would like to appeal. A sample letter is in Appendix C.) The form will ask you to briefly state why you think the original decision is wrong.

If the amount in question is less than $100, this will be your only opportunity to change the decision. It's therefore important that you give the carrier all the information you have that supports your case. If you think that a written statement from your doctor will help your appeal, now is the time to obtain it and send it to the carrier. Mail your request for reconsideration either to the intermediary or to your local Social Security office.

When your request for reconsideration is received, the intermediary will review its decision (called the initial determination). The intermediary will consider

1. all of the evidence it had when it made its initial determination

2. any new evidence you or others may present, and

3. any medical and other records that are found in the course of the reconsideration

Based on this review, the intermediary will issue a second decision (called a reconsidered determination). The reconsidered determination will either uphold or correct the intermediary's decision, give the reasons why, and advise you of your right to a hearing if more than $100 is in question.

Step 2: A Hearing Before an Administrative Law Judge

If the intermediary refuses to correct the initial decision (or if it makes some correction, but you are still dissatisfied), the next step is to request a hearing before an administrative law judge. You are entitled to a hearing only if the amount in question is over $100.

In most cases, the amount in question for an appeal will be equal to the charges found not to be covered, less any deductible and co-payment amounts. For example, if your claim for $892 for inpatient hospital services was denied, the amount in question would be ($892 − $592 [Hospital Insurance Deductible] = $300). This would be true whether or not you have paid the deductible. If there is any question about whether you meet the $100 minimum, request a hearing anyway. The judge will decide whether you meet the $100 minimum.

To request a hearing, fill out a Request for Hearing, Part A Hospital Insurance Benefits (Form HA 501.1) Mail the completed form to the intermediary or your local Social Security office within 60 days after you received the decision on your request for reconsideration.

When your request is received, your case will be assigned to an administrative law judge from the Social Security Administration. The judge will be responsible for gathering all of the evidence relevant to your appeal and for making a decision based on that evidence. When you request a hearing, the intermediary will automatically send your file to the law judge. The file should include all of the medical records on which the initial and reconsidered determinations were based.

The judge will set a time and place for the hearing. A typical hearing is usually informal, lasts about 20 to 30 minutes, and consists of a discussion between you and the judge. At the hearing, the judge will give you a chance to explain why you think Medicare should pay your claim. You also have the right to present witnesses and documents to support your case. Usually, no one from the intermediary will be there to oppose you. Their position is already on record.

If you think you will need some help at the hearing, ask a relative or friend to come with you. He or she can listen to what the judge has to say, take notes, and keep track of the points you want to bring to the judge's attention. In some cases (for example, if you are physically unable to go to the hearing), you may want to appoint someone to represent you. (For more information, see page 84.)

After the judge has received all of the evidence, he or she will send you a written decision either upholding or correcting the intermediary's decision. Simple cases are usually decided within 30 days of the hearing.

Step 3: The Social Security Appeals Council

If you believe that the judge's decision is incorrect, you can request that the Social Security Appeals Council review your case. To request a review, fill out a Request for Appeals Council Review of Hearing Decision (Form HA 520) and send it to your local Social Security office within 60 days after you have received the judge's decision.

After looking at your file, the Appeals Council will decide whether to grant a review. If the council decides to review your case, it may give you an opportunity to submit additional evidence, after which it will issue a decision. Getting help from the Appeals Council is a long shot, but you must appeal to the council if you intend to take your case to court.

Step 4: Filing a Lawsuit

If the Appeals Council denies your request for review, or grants review but issues an unsatisfactory decision, you may file a lawsuit in federal court. The suit must be filed within 60 days after you have received the Appeals Council decision, and the amount in question in your appeal must be over $1,000.

If a large amount of money or an important principle is at stake, you might decide that it is worthwhile to press your case in court. On more than one occasion, the government has dropped or changed a procedure that was grossly unfair to people on Medicare because a Medicare recipient was willing to stand up and challenge the practice in court.

If you go to court, however, you will need to be represented by an attorney. If there is a senior legal services program in your area, the program may be able to evaluate your case and represent you. If not, look to a local law school for help or seek a private attorney who specializes in Medicare cases.

HOW TO APPEAL A PART-B CLAIM

If the Medicare carrier denies all or part of a claim for doctors' services, outpatient services, or other services covered by Medical Insurance (Part B), you have up to five opportunities to change that decision.

Step 1: Review by the Carrier

The review stage is a good opportunity to correct relatively simple errors. Sometimes a carrier will deny a claim only because the provider left out a code on the itemized bill or used the wrong code. Sometimes a carrier will assume that a claim duplicates another billing, when in fact you received the same or similar services on more than one occasion and were billed separately for each. Mistakes like these are common. If you haven't done so already, ask the provider to help you with your appeal. The provider may be able to straighten things out simply by sending the insurance carrier some additional information.

The first step in appealing a denial of a Medicare Medical Insurance claim is to request that the carrier review your claim. Your request for review must be made within six months after your claim was denied. You can request a review no matter how much or how little your claim is for; just fill out a Request for Review of Part B Medicare Claim (Form HCFA 1964) and send it to the carrier or to your local Social Security office.

If the amount in question is less than $100, it's important that you submit all of the information that supports your case to the carrier at this time. This will be your only opportunity to change the carrier's decision.

When your request is received, the carrier will conduct a complete review of your claim. The review must be conducted by someone other than the person who made the initial determination. All of the evidence in the carrier's possession when it made the initial determination will be reviewed, as well as any new evidence you may want to present.

If, after reviewing the evidence, the carrier decides to pay the claim, it will send you a check and a new Explanation of Medical Benefits. The EOMB will state why the review determination is different from the initial determination. If the carrier decides that the initial determination is correct and that no additional payment should be made, it will send you a letter informing you of its decision and your right to request a hearing. Carriers are now required to complete all reviews within 45 days of receiving a request.

In 1987, carriers reviewed 5.5 million initial determinations under this procedure. Of this amount, 3.3 million, or 60 percent, were resolved either in whole or in part in favor of the person filing the claim.

Step 2: A Hearing Before a Hearing Officer

If the carrier refuses to change its initial determination and the amount in question is over $100, you can request a hearing for your Part-B claim before a hearing officer. You must make the request within six months of receiving the letter from the carrier upholding the initial determination. To request a hearing, fill out a Request for Hearing—Part B Medical Claim (HCFA 1965) and send it to the carrier or to your local Social Security office.

Upon receipt of your request for a hearing, the carrier will assign the case to a hearing officer. Hearing officers are usually attorneys who are knowledgeable about Medicare payment requirements. Although they are hired by the carrier, they are supposed to be impartial. After a case has been assigned, the carrier will transfer the file containing all of the information on your claim to the hearing officer.

The hearing must be held at a time and place that are reasonably convenient to you. In most cases, it will be held at the nearest Social Security office. If that is inconvenient, you can request that it be held at your home.

At the hearing, the officer will give you a chance to explain why you think Medicare should pay the claim. You also have the right to present witnesses and documents to support your case. A representative from the carrier may attend the hearing to answer questions from the hearing officer about how your claim was handled.

Based on the evidence received at the hearing, the hearing officer will prepare a written decision on your claim. Carriers are now required to issue these decisions within 120 days of receiving a request for a hearing. If the amount in question is less than $500, the hearing officer's decision is final.

In 1987, there were 48,366 hearings before carrier hearing officers. Of these, 22,189, or 46 percent, resulted in a total or partial victory for the person filing the claim.

Step 3: A Hearing Before an Administrative Law Judge

If you are dissatisfied with the hearing officer's decision, and the amount in question is over $500, you may request a hearing before an administrative law judge from the Social Security Administration. To request the hearing, fill out Request for Hearing (Form HA 501). The procedures for that hearing are the same as for hearings involving Hospital Insurance claims. (See pages 73 to 74.)

Step 4: An Appeal to the Social Security Appeals Council

If you are dissatisfied with the law judge's decision, your next step is to appeal to the Social Security Appeals Council. The procedure is the same as for appealing a Hospital Insurance claim. (See page 74.)

Step 5: Filing a Lawsuit

If the Appeals Council denies your appeal, and the amount in question is over $1,000, you can challenge the decision by filing a lawsuit in federal court. To take this step, you will need to be represented by an attorney. (See pages 74–75.)

HOW TO HANDLE YOUR OWN APPEAL

Except for the last step—going to court—you don't need a lawyer to represent you during an appeal. If you are handling your own appeal, here are some steps that will make your efforts more effective.

1. Getting Help from Your Doctor

If you decide to appeal, you will probably need some help from your doctor. Most appeals involve questions about a person's medical condition and how he or she was treated for that condition. The following kinds of questions may need to be answered: Did you need skilled nursing care? Were you actually confined to your home? Were the services of a second doctor really necessary, given your condition? Your doctor is in the best position to know the facts of your particular medical condition, to explain why Medicare should pay for the treatment you received, or to challenge the reasons given for denying your claim and show why they are wrong.

To support your appeal your doctor will need to prepare a written statement. In most cases, the doctor's statement is the single most important evidence in the appeal. The statement may be submitted in connection with either the request for review, or if the amount in question is more than $100, later at a hearing before a judge or hearing officer. While most doctors are too busy to attend a hearing, some will note the date and time for the hearing and make themselves available by telephone if the judge or hearing officer needs to ask them any direct questions.

Most doctors are willing to help their patients with an appeal, especially when their professional reputation and economic interest are at stake. When a carrier denies a claim, it often rejects the particular treatment that the doctor prescribed. Professional pride alone often causes doctors to vigorously defend their actions. In addition, most doctors know that if carriers refuse to pay legitimate claims, patients will soon be unable to afford their services. If your doctor is unwilling to help you with your appeal, consider looking for a new doctor.

2. Doing the Initial Research Required

Find out exactly why the intermediary or carrier denied your claim. If the intermediary or carrier relied on the advice of a consultant, be sure to get a copy of his or her report and a statement of qualifications. What particular fact or facts in those records did the intermediary or carrier consider important? Why were these facts important? What specific guidelines did it follow when it made its decision? The best way to get this information is to send a written request to the intermediary or carrier. This request can be made in connection with your initial request for reconsideration or request for review. (A sample letter appears in Appendix C.)

3. Preparing Your Case

After you understand why your claim was denied, begin developing your case. Write down exactly why you think your claim should have been paid. Avoid vague or emotional statements such as "denying the claim is unfair" or "I need the money." That might be true, but emotional appeals alone won't win your case. Instead, focus on how your claim fits the rules for Medicare payment. (For example: "My claim for home health services should have been paid because I was confined to my home and needed part-time, skilled nursing care for three weeks.") Rewrite your statement until it is as clear as possible.

Next, make a list of all of the witnesses, documents, and other evidence that would support your statement. For example, if your medical condition is an important issue, statements from your doctor and others who treated you would be important pieces of evidence. Hospital and other medical records may be useful in substantiating your condition. A friend or relative who visited you regularly could testify about what he or she observed.

Use your list in collecting the evidence you need. You may need to contact your doctor, track down the specialist who treated you, talk to the nurse who visited you at home, get copies of certain records, and obtain written statements. Add to the list if your research leads to other important sources of information.

In some cases, it might be helpful for the judge or hearing officer to actually see where you live or observe the services that you receive. For example, if your claim for home health services or durable medical equipment is denied, it might be useful for the hearing officer to see the kind of services delivered in your home, or how the equipment is actually used. If you believe that this kind of observation will be valuable, insist that the hearing be held at your home.

Before you make a final decision about what evidence to use, examine each item closely. What does a particular witness (document, record, etc.) add to your case? Could the evidence you plan to use hurt your case in any way, be confusing, or divert the decision maker's attention to an unimportant issue? Sort out whatever may be potentially harmful or superfluous. Be thorough and selective in preparing your case.

Once you have completed these preparations, you should be able to state exactly why Medicare should pay your claim and to point to the specific pieces of evidence you have to support your claim. For example:

> Medicare should pay for my home health care because I was confined to my home for three weeks after I returned from the hospital. During that time, I received skilled nursing care several hours a day, three days a week. The statements from my doctor and nurse, my hospital discharge record, the home health agency records, and testimony from my neighbor who came to visit me every day all show that I received this care and was in no condition to leave my home.

If you have difficulty writing your statement and gathering documentation on why Medicare should pay your claim, sit down with a friend or relative and examine your case together. By working together, the two of you may be able to arrive at a clear statement of what your case is all about and to develop ways to make it even stronger.

4. If You Don't Win Right Away

If you don't win your appeal right away, don't be discouraged. While some denials are reversed at the first step, your best chance of winning may be before the administrative law judge. Often, the judge is the only totally independent person who will examine your case. He or she is required to ensure that your appeal receives a fair and full hearing. If you don't win at an early stage, pursue your appeal to the law judge, and then make the most of that opportunity.

5. Protecting Your Right to a Hearing

If your claim is for more than the minimum amount, you have a right to a face-to-face hearing in front of a judge or hearing officer. The rules also allow for hearings to be conducted by telephone and for appeals to be decided entirely on the basis of written materials, but you must agree that these methods are acceptable to you. Intermediaries, carriers, and busy judges often favor these methods because they are less expensive and faster than traditional hearing procedures.

Keep in mind that these shortcuts may not be better for you. Under the conditions of a regular hearing, the judge or hearing officer has a chance to see and hear from you and your witnesses directly. In some cases, it may be important for him or her to see your physical condition rather than rely on descriptions of it.

If you think that a face-to-face hearing is important to your case, don't settle for something less. If you are asked to accept an alternative arrangement, refuse the offer. (Say, for example: "I know that holding a hearing where we can see each other face-to-face might mean that I will have to wait longer, but I'm more than willing to wait. I think that it's important for you to have the chance to actually see me and my witnesses. I don't believe that I will have a fair hearing unless that happens.")

The average waiting time for a hearing before an administrative law judge is about seven months. In some areas, you may need to wait up to six months for a hearing that is to be based only on written material, and up to one year for a face-to-face hearing.

6. Getting Ready for the Hearing

If you plan to present witnesses, be sure to prepare them for the hearing. Witnesses who are afraid, who tend to get on their favorite soapbox, or who fail to show up will be of no help to you. The best witness is one who is comfortable, responsive, alert, and on time.

A day or two before the hearing, take plenty of time to review the nature of the hearing with each witness. Let your witnesses know that the judge will probably ask them questions, and that these questions will be to gather information, not to cross-examine them. Remind them to listen to the questions carefully, to answer them as clearly and directly as possible, and to discuss only the subject related to the question the judge has asked. Review the information that you have asked the witness to testify to, and make certain that he or she is prepared to be clear about it.

Write down the date, time, and place for the hearing for your witnesses and make sure that they know how to get there. Arrange car pools or other transportation if necessary. Ask them to meet you at the hearing room at least ten minutes before it begins, just in case there are some last-minute items to discuss.

Before the hearing, make three copies of each document that you would like the judge to have: one for you and two for the judge. Make sure that all of the copies are legible and complete. Bring all three copies to the hearing and organize them so that you can refer to them easily. Make a list of all the witnesses and documents you plan to present, and bring the list to the hearing.

Look over anything the insurance carrier might present to support its original decision. Carriers will often submit a written statement by their "medical consultant" about your claim. The consultant is usually a doctor who is an employee of the carrier. These consultants often express opinions on subjects about which they have little or no expertise. For example, a doctor who has no training or experience in treating arthritis might criticize or otherwise disparage the services you received from a specialist. If that's true, make a note to point out that fact at the hearing.

7. At the Hearing

Arrive early. When the hearing begins, the judge will explain how he or she plans to conduct it. Usually, the judge will ask you whether you plan to present any witnesses or documents. Tell him or her how many witnesses you have and briefly describe the documents you would like to present.

Before the hearing is concluded, check your list to make sure that the judge has received all of the documents and heard from all of your witnesses. If you are not sure whether the judge has a certain document, ask.

During a hearing, events often happen differently from the way you had planned. A judge might ask for one document before the others, or might seem especially interested in hearing from one particular witness, or spend more time than you expected on a specific point, or simply call a break at an unexpected time. When things like this happen, it's easy to get flustered and forget to present the other documents, call the other witnesses, or bring up the rest of the points you feel are important. For this reason, it's a good idea to ask someone to help you at the hearing. Choose a friend or relative who is calm, well organized, and will give you good moral support. Ask that person to keep your documents organized and to quietly remind you if you forget a witness, document, or anything else that's important to your case. Also, ask this associate to note anything that you promise to send the judge, and the date by which the judge must receive it.

If, at the end of the hearing, you believe that there is some additional evidence that would be helpful, ask the judge if you can send in that evidence. For example, it may be important for your doctor to clarify something in his or her statement, or to address an issue that the statement did not cover. Most judges will agree to your request.

8. Meeting Deadlines

At each stage of the appeals process, there is a deadline for taking the next step. To appeal a denial of a Medical Insurance claim, for example, you must send in a Request for Review within six months of receiving the notice of denial. Mark these deadlines on your calendar and take all steps to meet them. Missing a deadline could mean the end of your appeal, even if you have a good case.

APPOINTING SOMEONE TO REPRESENT YOU

If you prefer it, you are allowed to appoint someone to represent you in an appeal. That person could be anyone you trust, such as a spouse, a son or daughter, another close relative, or a friend, attorney, or social worker. Both you and the person you select as a representative must complete an Appointment of Representative form (Form HCFA1696). The form should be mailed to the agency you are currently appealing to.

Once the form is received, your representative will be able to act on your behalf. He or she can receive notices, request information, and present evidence. In short, your representative will be able to do everything you can in connection with the appeal.

If a person is unable to pursue an appeal because of death or impairment, the legal representative of the estate or the custodian may appeal for that person. If you are serving in that capacity, explain that you are acting on the person's behalf when you submit a request for review or reconsideration.

9

How to Cope
with Problem Bills

BILLS THAT YOU DON'T HAVE TO PAY

If your Medicare claim is denied, you are usually responsible for paying the entire bill. For example, if your doctor sends you a bill for $500 and Medicare denies the claim, you are normally responsible for paying your doctor the entire $500. Despite this general rule, there are a few instances in which you are *not* obligated to pay the bill.

Problems with Assigned Claims

In certain categories, the Medicare intermediary or carrier will determine whether you or the provider of your health-care services "knew or should have known whether the services would be covered" when an assigned claim is denied. The answer to this question will determine who pays for the services. These categories are:

1. The services were not covered because they were custodial in nature.

2. Home health services were not covered because either you weren't confined to your home or you didn't require intermittent skilled nursing care.

3. The services were not reasonable and necessary.

If the intermediary or carrier finds that *neither you nor the provider* knew, or should have known, that the services would not be covered, then Medicare pays for the services as if they were covered. If it finds that the *provider knew,* or should have known, that Medicare would not pay for the services, the provider is liable for the bill. You are under no obligation to pay the provider. But if the carrier or intermediary finds that *you knew,* or should have known, that the services were not covered, you are responsible for paying the entire bill. Here are some examples of how these rules work.

When Medicare Pays the Bill

Doctor X performs an operation under Medicare assignment and submits a claim to the Medicare insurance carrier. The carrier reviews the claim and determines that the operation was not reasonable and necessary; the day before the operation, new regulations were issued and that operation is now considered obsolete. The carrier finds that because of lack of notice, neither you nor your doctor knew, or should have known, that Medicare would not pay for the operation. Therefore, even though the operation is not technically covered by Medicare, the carrier will pay for it as if it were covered. You are still responsible for paying the deductible and the 20 percent co-payment.

When the Doctor Foots the Bill

In a second situation, the facts are the same as in the example just mentioned, except that three months before your operation, the Medicare carrier mailed a notice to all doctors in the state, including Doctor X, informing them that the operation would no longer be covered as of a certain date. Based on this notice, the carrier finds that Doctor X knew, or should have known, that Medicare would not pay for the operation.

In this case, the doctor will have to absorb the entire cost of the services. The carrier will refuse to pay the claim and inform you in the EOMB that you are under no obligation to pay. The doctor has the right to appeal the carrier's decision.

If you already have paid the doctor, you will need to file a "request for indemnification." (A Social Security office or your carrier can help you.) After you file your request, the carrier will refund the money you paid the provider and deduct that amount from a future payment it makes to the provider.

WHEN YOU PAY THE BILL

In yet another situation, the facts are the same as in the previous example, except that a month before the operation, Doctor X gave you written notice that the operation would not be covered by Medicare, and you agreed in writing to pay the entire bill if Medicare refused to pay. Based on the notice you received, the carrier finds that you knew, or should have known, that Medicare would not pay. In this case, the carrier will refuse to pay the claim, and you are responsible for paying the full amount to Doctor X. You can appeal the decision if the notice and the agreement are either vague or a forgery, or if you believe that the doctor tricked or coerced you into signing the agreement to pay.

PROBLEMS WITH UNASSIGNED CLAIMS

If a doctor who does not accept Medicare assignment provides you with services, and if Medicare subsequently denies your claim because it finds that these services were not medically necessary, you may be entitled to a refund. Again, this will be determined when and if the Medicare carrier finds that the doctor knew, or should have known, that the services would not be covered. But no refund is required if the doctor notified you of any likelihood that Medicare would not pay for the specific service, and, after being notified, you agreed to pay for the service.

Medicare guidelines require that the physician's advance notice to the patient must (1) clearly identify the particular service, (2) state that the physician believes that Medicare is likely to deny payment for the particular service, and (3) give the physician's reason(s) for his or her belief that Medicare is likely to deny payment. Because of these requirements, none of the following procedures can allow physicians to avoid their obligation to make refunds: (1) requiring patients to sign a blanket agreement consenting to pay for all services denied by Medicare, (2) sending out routine notices to patients stating that Medicare denials are a possibility, or (3) telling patients personally that they never know when Medicare will deny a claim. The notice to you must have been specific, or the claim will be denied.

Let's assume, for example, that you are treated by Dr. Y, who does not accept Medicare assignment. You pay Dr. Y $1,000 for the services he provided and then you submit a claim to the Medicare carrier. On reviewing the claim, the carrier decides that Dr. Y's services were not medically necessary.

The carrier will send you an EOMB denying your claim and notifying you of your right to a refund from Dr. Y. (You may have to look hard for this notice, because it often comes near the end of the EOMB and may be presented with other information.) At the same time, the carrier will also send a notice to the doctor.

Dr. Y will have 30 days to either refund your money or request a review of the carrier's decision. If a review is requested and no changes are made, the doctor must refund the money within 15 days of the review decision.

These rules also apply to situations where the carrier pays a reduced amount because it finds that the doctor's services were more extensive than necessary. If the doctor knew, or should have known, that Medicare would not pay for the more extensive services and did not tell you before providing the services, you are entitled to a refund of any amount you paid that is more than the amount for these services approved by the carrier. Let's assume, for example, that you also paid Dr. Y $150 for an extensive office visit. The carrier concludes that an extensive visit was not necessary and reasonable, and it pays you only $80, based on the Medicare-approved charge for a routine visit of $100. You are entitled to a refund from Dr. Y of $50.

WHEN THE BILLS ARE MORE
THAN YOU CAN AFFORD TO PAY

After Medicare and whatever private insurance you may retain have paid their designated share of the bills, there usually will be an amount left for you to pay. If the amount is more than you can afford to pay, taking the following steps might help to bring down the amount to a level you can afford, or even eliminate it entirely. Here are a few examples of how some seniors have addressed the problem of big bills:

Mrs. S, a recent widow, was billed $1,200 in doctors' fees for medical treatment for her late husband. With help from a senior advocate, she found that the services were considered medically unnecessary. By law, the doctor could not charge her for those services. The advocate assisted her in having the bills withdrawn entirely.

On reviewing bills from his physician, Mr. A found that he was being overcharged by $20 per visit. The doctor, who had agreed to accept Medicare assignment, did not know that it was illegal to charge Mr. A more than the Medicare-approved amount. When this was brought to the attention of his office staff, a series of more reasonable charges was issued.

Mr. and Mrs. C were facing huge expenses for doctors, laboratory tests, and X rays. They asked each provider to lower its bills to the amount that Medicare and their supplemental policy would pay. All but one agreed, and that provider allowed Mr. and Mrs. C to pay its fees in installments of $20 per month.

1. Review Your Bills

Despite receiving regular notices from Medicare, some providers bill seniors for more than the law allows. You are not obligated to pay illegal charges, and you should not do so. If you have already paid the provider, you are entitled to a refund. Review your bills to find out:

If doctors charged you more than the Medicare-approved amount. Doctors who accept assignment may charge only the Medicare-approved amount for their services. Since Medicare will pay eighty percent of that amount directly to the doctor, you should pay only 20 percent of the approved amount after meeting the annual deductible. There should be no other charges. (For more information about Medicare assignment, see Chapter 2.)

Doctors who don't accept assignment are allowed to charge you higher rates for most services. The law now requires that they give you a prior, written notice of their charges for any elective surgery over $500. Elective surgery is basically any surgery that can be scheduled in advance or that can be delayed without a risk of death or permanent impairment. The notice from your physician must state the estimated charge for the surgery, how much Medicare will pay, and how much you will have to pay. If your doctor does not give you the required notice, he or she cannot charge you more than the Medicare-approved amount. If you have already paid more, you're entitled to a refund. Beginning in 1992, doctors who do not accept Medicare assignment are prohibited from charging fees that are more than 15 percent above the Medicare-approved amount.

If doctors charged for unnecessary or unreasonable services. Whether your doctor accepts Medicare assignment or not, you do not have to pay for services that Medicare considers unnecessary or unreasonable. If Medicare denies a claim for that reason, the doctor may charge you for those services only if you were informed in advance that Medicare would not pay for them *and* you agreed in writing to pay for them.

To find out whether any of the services billed fall into this category, examine your Explanation of Medical Benefits. The EOMB will give a reason for each claim Medicare denies. For services Medicare considers to have been unnecessary, the EOMB might state either "the service is not reasonable and necessary" or simply "not a covered service." If the latter reason appears on your EOMB, call the carrier's toll-free number (printed at the top of the EOMB) to find out whether the service was considered unnecessary.

If providers overcharged for clinical lab services. When a doctor or laboratory accepts assignment, clinical laboratory services performed by that provider are paid in full by Medicare. You should not be billed at all for these services. You cannot be billed an amount over the Medicare-approved amount, and unlike other services, there is no 20 percent co-payment requirement for clinical laboratory services.

If you find any of these illegal charges on your bill, point them out to the provider and write to insist that they be removed. (See sample letter in Appendix C.) If you have already paid the provider, request that it refund your money within 30 days. If the provider refuses or ignores your request, inform your Medicare carrier and one or more of the law enforcement agencies listed in Appendix B. (A sample letter to such a law enforcement agency appears in Appendix C.) In addition, report the problem to the inspector general of the U.S. Department of Health and Human Services. This department maintains a Fraud and Abuse Hotline to receive complaints concerning illegal charges by providers. The toll-free numbers are: 800-368-5779 and 800-638-3986.

2. Double-check All Sources of Payment

Make sure you have not overlooked any health insurance source for paying the bills. Check whether you have submitted claims to Medicare and to any additional insurers that pay for portions of your medical expenses. Have all of the claims been processed? If any claims are still outstanding, call your Medicare carrier or your supplementary or other health insurance company to find out the status of your claim. Follow up and resolve any problems.

3. Negotiate with Providers

If the charges that you cannot afford to pay are found to be proper, try to get the health-care provider to agree to either write off part of the bill or to receive payment in small monthly installments. This may take some preparation.

Before you contact the provider, prepare a simple budget. Start with your monthly income and subtract your monthly expenses for food, housing, utilities, insurance, and other essentials. This budget will give you a realistic idea of how much is left over to pay outstanding bills. Use it to guide your negotiations with the doctor or other providers.

Many doctors refuse to discuss problems concerning billing, and direct patients to a bookkeeper, office manager, or a billing department. Depending on the doctor's bill-collection policies, the person you are directed to may be formidable and intimidating or sympathetic. Be prepared to be firm and pleasantly tenacious.

When you reach the right person, explain the situation. ("I understand that Medicare and my insurance have paid their share of these bills, and there is still a balance of $ ____ owing on my account. I'm calling because I cannot afford to pay that amount.") The budget you have prepared will help you explain why you are unable to pay. ("My monthly income, including Social Security, is only $ ____, and most of that goes for rent, food, utilities, and insurance. My savings were spent on paying the bills from my last illness.")

The next question to ask is whether the provider will consider lowering the bill. ("Would Dr. ____ reduce the amount to something I could afford?") Don't be quick to give in if the answer is an immediate no. If it is, ask if the provider would agree to receive installment payments over an extended period of time. ("I can't pay that amount in one lump sum, but I could pay $ ____ every month.") Add that you hope the doctor will be able to waive any finance charges during that period.

Be persistent. The initial responses may not be encouraging, but stick to your position. You may have to say the same thing several times before the person you are speaking with is convinced that some kind of adjustment is needed. ("I'm sorry, but it's really not possible for me to pay that amount." "After paying for rent, food, and utilities, I can only afford to pay you $ ____ a month." "I just don't have that much money.")

Even if you feel embarrassed or pressured, don't agree to something you cannot afford. Paying a $350 doctor's bill and then having your utilities turned off, for example, is not a good solution. Sometimes, it may take several discussions to arrive at a payment you can afford. Even if the possibilities seem dim, try to keep the topic open. ("Please consider what I've said. I would like to arrange for something I can afford, and I'll call the office again at the end of the week to see how we can work this out.")

Before you accept or reject any payment plan, consider the options that are available in your community. If you live in a large city with easy access to many health-care providers, you may be freer to negotiate than if you live in a rural area where other providers may be many miles away. In the latter case, you may feel that it is so important to maintain good relations with your present providers that you are willing to risk financial consequences elsewhere to satisfy the demand for payment.

Negotiating, particularly over bills, can be a highly emotional process. Guilt, shame, and pressure are only a few of the tactics used by some health-care providers, or those acting for them, to collect delinquent accounts. Unless you are skillful at dealing with such tactics, consider asking someone you trust to act for you. You need a person who can be objective and persistent, and who can communicate clearly—perhaps a relative, a friend, or an advocate from a local seniors' program.

One cautionary note for children and other relatives: doctors, hospital administrators, or other providers may ask you to take responsibility for some or all of the outstanding bill. *Do not automatically agree to do so. In most cases, you are under no legal obligation to pay those bills.* About half of the states have repealed laws requiring that adult children help support their parents. In states where such laws are still on the books, courts have rarely enforced them. Because assuming the responsibility for large medical bills may impose considerable hardship on you and your family, try to find other solutions. If necessary, get advice from a senior legal services or senior counseling program in your area. (See Appendix B.)

MEDICAID

Some bills may be so large that, despite all efforts, they drain nearly all of your financial resources. If you are in that situation, you might be eligible for Medicaid, the government program that pays for medical services for low-income persons of all ages.

The rules for qualifying for Medicaid and the benefits offered vary from state to state. In general, a person qualifies for Medicaid if he or she is eligible for public assistance or Supplementary Security Income (SSI). Paying large medical bills is one way a person may become eligible for these programs.

In every state, the services covered by Medicaid include inpatient and outpatient hospital services, skilled nursing care, doctors' services, home health services, and lab and X-ray services. In some states, Medicaid will cover additional services such as podiatrist services, eyeglasses, dental care, and prescription drugs.

To find out whether you qualify for Medicaid and what specific services are covered in your state, contact your local public assistance, social services, or welfare office. You will be asked to fill out a detailed application listing your assets, income, and expenses. In addition, someone from the agency may interview you.

If you are found eligible, Medicaid will pay for services by providers who have agreed to accept Medicaid patients and Medicaid's payment as payment in full. Medicaid will pay for services from participating providers as far back as three months before the date you apply. Participating providers will be paid directly by Medicaid, and they cannot bill you extra for covered services. Ask your current doctors whether they accept Medicaid. If they do not, ask them to refer you to doctors who do.

If you meet both programs' eligibility requirements, you can receive benefits from Medicare and Medicaid at the same time. In that case, Medicare will pay for covered services first, and then

Medicaid will pay for deductibles, co-payments, and certain services not covered by Medicare.

If your income and assets are low but not low enough to qualify for Medicaid, your state may pay for your Medicare premiums and for some of the deductibles and co-payments as well. The requirements in 1989 were that your annual income be less than $5,770 ($7,730 for a couple) and your assets, not including your home, must be less than $4,000. If you think you might qualify, contact your state or local welfare, social service, or public health office.

Many older people who have led productive lives find it painful to apply for government assistance even when they desperately need it. If you find that you need help, don't be reluctant to get the benefits to which you are entitled. Medicaid and other government programs are part of the public safety net that you helped establish and pay for.

Where to Go for Help

Problems from large bills can come in many forms, including aggressive bill collectors, threatening letters, and unsympathetic health-care providers. Many people try to deal with these problems alone, without realizing that competent help is available in their community.

A growing number of states have health insurance counseling services specifically for senior citizens. These programs help seniors make sense of their bills, file claims, deal with health-care providers, and apply for Medicaid. When legal help is needed, they refer cases to senior legal services programs or district attorneys. To find out whether a health insurance counseling program exists in your area, contact your state office on aging. (For more information, see Appendix B.)

10

Long-term Care

When Medicare was first enacted, Congress assumed that its typical beneficiary would be a person who was sick or injured and needed to be hospitalized for a short time; then, it was assumed, he or she would return home to resume a normal life. While some Medicare patients conform to this example, many do not. Conditions such as Alzheimer's disease, arthritis, and stroke often leave a permanent disability or lead to a long period of supervision and care.

Despite this common necessity for long-term health care, there is no coordinated system in place for providing that care to older people. As a result, older people and their families bear much of the burden when it comes to finding and paying for these services.

WHO NEEDS LONG-TERM CARE?

People need long-term care when a physical or mental disability prevents them from being able to take care of themselves. Disabled persons may need help with everyday activities such as bathing, dressing, eating, getting to the toilet, or moving from a bed or chair. To enable them to live at home, they may also need help with shopping, cooking, or housework. Currently, more than 9 million Americans of all ages require this kind of help. More than half of them are elderly.

The likelihood of a person becoming disabled increases with age. For people between the ages of 65 and 74, fewer than one out of seven are disabled. This number increases to two in seven for those between the ages of 75 and 84. For seniors above age 85, four out of seven are disabled.

Most of the long-term care needed by older disabled people is provided at home by spouses, children, and other family members. Much of this care is provided seven days a week. About one-fourth of the disabled elderly live in nursing homes, while approximately three-fourths live in the community.

WHAT KINDS OF SERVICES ARE AVAILABLE?

For years, long-term care meant only one thing: nursing homes. Fortunately, the situation is changing. Increasingly, older people and their families are able to choose from a range of long-term care services based on their individual needs. In many communities, there now are services that permit disabled seniors to live safely and comfortably at home. The following are only some of the services that help people who need long-term care:

Homemaker Services

Homemakers are people employed to help older people who are able to live at home but have difficulty with household tasks such as cleaning, cooking, food shopping, and laundry. Receiving homemaker help with these simple but essential jobs can mean the difference between living at home or going to a nursing home.

Adult Day Care

Adult day-care programs help people with jobs care for an elderly parent or spouse who needs constant supervision by providing that supervision during working hours. Usually, the elderly parent or spouse is dropped off at the adult day-care center in the morning and picked up at the end of the day. These programs often provide other services, such as recreation, nutrition, rehabilitation, and transportation.

Adult Foster Care

Adult foster-care programs place older persons who need personal care with families in private homes. The homes are usually licensed by the state, and the families are paid a fee for the supervision and care they provide. Foster care allows older persons without relatives to remain in the community.

Respite Care

Respite-care programs support spouses, children, and others who care for an elderly person at home by providing time off for vacations or personal needs. Some respite programs place elderly persons in a nursing home for a short time, while others train and pay people to provide short-term care at the elderly person's home.

Hospice Care

Hospice programs are specially designed to provide care to people who are dying. These programs help assure that patients are as comfortable and free of pain as possible and include counseling for both patients and survivors. Hospice services can be provided at home or in a special hospice facility.

Home Health Care

Home health care programs bring nurses, rehabilitation therapists, home health aides, and other trained people into homes to provide care to homebound patients. The level of care can range from basic help with getting in and out of bed, bathing, and taking medications to the use of sophisticated medical equipment. When used with other services, home health care allows older persons to live for years at home even if they are in declining health. This kind of care is often arranged through private home health agencies that hire home health workers.

Nursing Home Care

Nursing homes are facilities where people who cannot care for themselves live and receive various kinds of care. They are sometimes called convalescent hospitals, nursing centers, geriatric centers, retirement homes, rest homes, and residential care centers. Three levels of care are available in nursing homes, though often not in the same facility: skilled nursing care, intermediate care, and custodial care.

In many states, "convalescent hospitals" are skilled nursing facilities that provide short-term, recuperative care to patients. They may or may not qualify for Medicare reimbursement, depending on whether they meet Medicare standards and have applied for eligibility. Some nursing homes that could qualify have chosen not to apply.

Skilled Nursing Care

Skilled nursing care is the highest level of care, similar in many ways to the degree of care provided in a hospital. In a skilled nursing facility (SNF), care is provided to patients on a daily basis by licensed nurses or licensed therapists under the direction of a doctor. This type of care might include intravenous injections, changing sterile dressings, and physical, occupational, or speech therapy.

Patients in skilled nursing facilities are usually recovering from an acute illness or have serious chronic medical problems. If they improve or no longer benefit from skilled nursing care, they are placed in intermediate care or sent home.

Intermediate Nursing Care

Intermediate nursing care provides less intensive medical care than skilled care. The services provided are still rendered regularly by licensed professionals, but not on a daily basis. Patients receiving intermediate nursing care usually still need a substantial amount of personal care.

Custodial Care

Patients who need custodial care need personal rather than medical care. They may need help in getting in and out of bed, walking, eating, and bathing. In a health-related facility (HRF), custodial care can be provided by persons with less training than those providing skilled or intermediate care.

Nursing homes may provide more than one level of care at the same facility. For example, some nursing homes are licensed to provide both skilled nursing care and intermediate care. Patients may go from one level to another as their conditions change. Some nursing homes provide only custodial care. They are sometimes called board-and-care facilities, sheltered care facilities, or group homes. Often, they are affiliated with a facility that provides skilled or intermediate care.

Life Care Centers

Life care centers provide both living facilities and medical care to residents. Usually, residents live in apartments or cottages and receive care when necessary from a skilled nursing facility on the same premises. Some life care centers provide dining facilities, transportation, recreation, counseling, and other services. Unlike those who become residents of nursing homes, people move to life care centers when they are still healthy. Some centers have strict entrance requirements involving lengthy applications, health evaluations, and waiting periods before pre-existing conditions will be covered by the services provided.

Most life care centers charge substantial entrance fees in addition to monthly payments. According to a 1986 study, entrance fees of about $50,000 per person and monthly fees of $750 for a one-bedroom apartment were average. Some centers provide nursing-home care and other health services at no extra charge, but others charge regular fees for these services.

LICENSING, CERTIFICATION, AND ACCREDITATION

Providers of long-term care services may be "licensed," "certified," or "accredited." Each of these terms means something different:

- If a facility is *licensed*, it means that the facility has met certain minimum legal standards set by a state or local government agency. If the facility fails to meet those standards, it could be fined or, in an extreme case, ordered to close.

- A facility may also be *certified* by Medicare and/or Medicaid. This means that it meets the minimum standards for those programs and has agreed to accept Medicare and/or Medicaid patients. Medicare will only pay for care provided by Medicare-certified facilities, and Medicaid will only pay for care provided by Medicaid-certified facilities.

- A facility may also be *accredited* by an association. For example, some nursing homes are accredited by the American Association of Homes for the Aging. Accreditation means that the facility meets the standards set by an industry trade association. If the facility falls below those standards, usually the only consequence is loss of its membership in the association.

Do not rely solely on the fact that a facility is licensed, certified, or accredited in making your decision about whether it provides good care. None of these will guarantee that you will receive high-quality care. Because of tight budgets, enforcement of official licensing and certification standards is often spotty, and in matters of accreditation there is little that a trade association can actually do to enforce its voluntary standards. Beware of endorsements or façades: you will need to make your own on-premises evaluation of a long-term care facility.

HOW TO FIND SERVICES IN YOUR COMMUNITY

In most communities, nursing-home care, home health care, adult day care, homemaking assistance, and other services for long-term care are not well coordinated. As a result, individual families must do most of the work of finding, screening, and overseeing services. This responsibility often falls on a son or daughter, in-law, or the spouse of the person who needs care. Help in locating long-term care can be obtained through the following people and organizations. In every case, be sure to ask how recently the information you are offered has been updated;

a new administration at a facility can considerably improve or deteriorate the quality of the care provided.

Hospital Social Workers

If you or the family member who needs long-term care is a patient in the hospital, consult a hospital social worker about what long-term care facilities are available and appropriate. Once the level of care that you or your relative needs is determined, whoever is acting as your personal advocate—a relative or friend—in negotiating your health care can visit each recommended facility and make a personal assessment of the care provided and the atmosphere. Hospitals are often the best places from which to be referred to a long-term care facility, as hospital patients often are given priority over other applicants. This is not because of the urgency of the patients' conditions but because hospitals need occupied beds for new patients. As a result, hospitals can often negotiate prompt acceptance at facilities to which they are accustomed to referring patients. But be aware that this same incentive can cause hospitals to place patients in facilities that provide substandard care or care that is inappropriate for patients' conditions.

Doctors

If you or your relative is not hospitalized, doctors often can help you identify the kind of care that is needed and refer you to facilities and agencies that have experience in providing that care. Use those references, as well as any recent similar experiences of relatives and friends, as a starting point in your search.

Agencies on Aging

Under the Older Americans Act, the federal government distributes funds to state agencies on aging. These funds are used by local agencies on aging to support a wide variety of programs that assist people who need long-term care. The services include home health care, Meals-On-Wheels, transportation, and homemaking services. In addition, these agencies can direct you to other long-term care services in your area.

Agencies on aging are listed in the telephone directory, usually under local government services. You can also contact the agency on aging for your state. (See Appendix B for the name and number of the local agency in your area.)

Social Services Agencies

Many communities and nonprofit or religious organizations employ professionals who specialize in helping older people locate needed services. These professionals can help direct you to appropriate facilities, identify community resources, and cut through bureaucratic red tape. Regardless of the agency's title, you don't need to be on welfare or to practice a particular religion to get help.

To contact these agencies, consult your telephone directory under local government listings (Elderly Assistance, or Senior Citizens Assistance), individual listings (American Red Cross, Catholic Charities, Family Service Agency, Jewish Family [or Community] Services, Lutheran Social Services, and other such religious denominations), and Yellow Pages listings (Senior Citizens Service Organizations or Social Service Organizations).

Independent Social Workers and Geriatric Consultants

The business of seniors' finances and of locating good long-term care facilities has become so complex that in some communities experienced social workers have established independent practices that specialize exclusively in these matters. A single consultation, though expensive, could save you weeks of tedious investigation. Attorneys who specialize in the finances of seniors might be able to refer you to such an independent consultant. Especially in large cities, where a great number of long-term care facilities are available, such a consultation can be invaluable.

HOW TO SELECT A FACILITY

A social worker, doctor, agency on aging, or social services organization can direct you to facilities in your community, but you still need to use your own judgment in making a final decision. Before you select a home health agency, adult day-care program, nursing home, or life care center, investigate it thoroughly to make sure that it meets your needs.

If you are considering an adult day-care program, nursing home, or life care center, it is important that you or your advocate visit the facility. During the visit, check whether the facility is in a location that is safe and convenient (for drop-offs, visits, shopping, etc.).

Make sure that the premises are safe and habitable. Pay attention to whether there are smoke detectors, fire extinguishers, automatic sprinklers, and emergency exits. Check whether the walkways are clear and well maintained and whether the facilities and grounds are easily accessible to people in wheelchairs. Visit the living areas to see whether they are clean, neat, and arranged to provide enough privacy.

Spend some time quietly observing the staff. Check whether there seem to be enough trained people to provide quality care and whether the staff seems caring, friendly, and respectful toward the people they are caring for. If you visit a number of facilities, you will find that staff are generally sparse even in the best of them. Belt-tightening by Medicare and other government programs has caused many facilities to cut back their staff to minimum levels. With this general condition in mind, observe the people being cared for to see whether they are comfortable talking to the staff or asking for help. Insofar as their medical conditions allow it, they should be out of their rooms, dressed, and interested in what is going on rather than bored, withdrawn, or sleeping.

Find out what kinds of social, educational, or recreational activities are planned for the day. (There should be a calendar of activities available for the week or month.) If meals are served, visit the kitchen to make sure that it is clean. If you can, observe a meal to find out whether the patients are served at a reasonable time and in a pleasant place. Check whether the meal service is well organized and if the residents are given enough time to eat and socialize. Be sure that the food looks fresh and appetizing and is served at the right temperature. If possible, taste it yourself. Ask for a copy of that day's menu and of the menus planned for the next several weeks. From the menus, you should be able to determine whether there is enough choice and variety in what people are served. Find out whether the kitchen can accommodate special needs and diets.

If you can, make several visits to the facility at different times of the day. Each visit will give you more information about what the facility has to offer and whether it will meet your needs.

For some people, visiting a nursing home can be a distressing experience. If you feel that you would be too upset to ask the necessary questions or assess the nursing home objectively, ask someone you trust to visit the home for you. Have them review this chapter before the visit and later tell you what they learned.

Once you have narrowed the field to considering particular nursing homes or life care facilities, get copies of the latest inspection reports from your state or local health department. Those reports will tell you when the facilities were last inspected and what problems, if any, were found. In some states, these reports must also be posted on the premises.

Be sure to check whether the facility is certified by Medicare and/or Medicaid. Medicare will pay for care only from Medicare-certified providers. Medicaid will pay for care only from Medicaid-certified providers.

Checking Medicaid certification is particularly important if you are considering a nursing home. Even if you don't qualify for Medicaid now, you may need to look to Medicaid in the future. If the nursing home does not meet Medicaid standards or does not participate in Medicaid, you will need to move to another facility once your financial resources are depleted.

Find out what kind of experience, training, and licenses staff members have, and whether there is regular supervision of the staff. Also find out what arrangements the staff has made for medical emergencies. (For example, have arrangements been made with nearby hospitals for emergency care? Is there either a doctor on the premises or one that the staff can call in the event of an accident or sudden illness?) This information will help you determine whether the people responsible for providing care are qualified and have given adequate attention to critical items.

Be sure you understand the services an agency or facility provides and when those services are available. For example, there will be a problem if you need home health services seven days a week but the agency you are considering is closed on weekends.

Be sure that you understand all of the fees, including entrance fees, deposits, monthly fees, and fees for specific services. Some facilities have lower fees for people with lower incomes. Find out how often fees are raised and by how much.

11

Paying
for Long-term Care

Each year, Americans spend approximately $50 billion for long-term care. Nearly three-fourths of this goes for care in nursing homes. Most of this amount is paid by disabled people and their families.

Currently, the average annual cost of nursing-home care is about $25,000. Of the approximately $41 billion we spend for nursing-home care each year, nursing-home residents and their families pay for about 51 percent; Medicaid, on behalf of poor patients, pays 42 percent; other government programs, such as the Veterans Administration, pay 5 percent; Medicare pays slightly over one percent; and private insurance pays less than one percent.

Depending on the degree of disability, average annual expenses for paid home care can range from approximately $1,000 to $9,000. Some conditions, such as Alzheimer's disease, may cost substantially more. Of the $9 billion we spend annually for paid home care, 36 percent is paid by Medicare, 14 percent by Medicaid, 31 percent by other government programs (including the Veterans Administration and programs under the Older Americans Act), and 19 percent by disabled persons and their families.

These figures do not include the millions of hours of unpaid home care provided by families and friends. Three out of four disabled elderly live in the community, where they are cared for by their children, spouses, in-laws, grandchildren, other relatives, and friends. In many cases, care is provided seven days a week without the help of any paid services. Most families turn to nursing homes only as a last resort, when the physical, emotional, and financial burdens of caring for an elderly relative at home become too difficult for the family or care provider to manage.

WHAT MEDICARE WILL PAY FOR

The only long-term care services Medicare will pay for are

1. care in a Medicare-certified skilled nursing facility
2. part-time or intermittent home health services
3. hospice care

You should not rely on Medicare to meet either nursing-home or home health expenses on a long-term basis. In both cases, while the type of care covered is medically intense, the coverage extends only to relatively short-term care that is provided to help people recuperate from an illness or injury.

Skilled Nursing-Home Care

Medicare will pay for care in a skilled nursing home only if the following requirements are met:

1. You must have been hospitalized for at least three consecutive days and transferred to the nursing home within 30 days of leaving the hospital.
2. The nursing care must be provided in a skilled nursing facility that is certified by Medicare.
3. You must need skilled nursing care or physical, speech, or occupational therapy on a daily basis.
4. Care must be provided under a doctor's orders by (or under the supervision of) registered professional nurses and/or licensed therapists.

If you meet each of these requirements, Medicare will pay for up to 100 days of care for each spell of illness. It will pay the full cost of care for the first 20 days. For days 21 to 100, you are responsible for a co-payment of $74 per day (in 1990). After 100 days, you are responsible for the full amount.

Remember, skilled nursing care is the highest level of care, and not all nursing homes are Medicare-certified skilled nursing facilities. Medicare will *not* pay for lower levels of nursing-home care, nor will it pay for skilled care in a facility that is not Medicare-certified. To find out whether a facility is certified, check with the director of the facility or with your state agency on aging. (See Appendix B.)

Part-time or Intermittent Home Health Care

Medicare covers skilled nursing care, rehabilitation care, and other health-care services at home under certain conditions. To qualify, you must meet all of the following requirements:

1. You must be confined to your home.
2. You must be under the care of a doctor.
3. The doctor must establish a written plan for home health care that includes skilled nursing care on a part-time or intermittent basis, or physical or speech therapy.
4. The care must be provided by a Medicare-certified home health agency.

If you meet these four requirements, Medicare will pay for skilled nursing care and services of home health aides on a *part-time or intermittent basis*. It will also pay for physical, speech, or occupational therapy. Medicare will pay 100 percent of the cost of these services. No deductibles or co-payments are required.

"Part-time or intermittent" usually means for a few hours a day, several days a week, although in exceptional circumstances more care may be permitted for a short time. Medicare will not pay if you need full-time skilled care at home for an extended period of time, nor will it pay if you need only custodial care or homemaking services.

Hospice Care

Medicare will pay for up to 210 days of hospice care if the following requirements are met:

1. A doctor must certify that you are terminally ill.

2. You must choose to receive care from a hospice program instead of the regular Medicare benefits for the terminal illness. This means stopping curative treatment.

3. The care must be provided by a Medicare-certified hospice program.

If these requirements are met, Medicare will pay for nearly all of your expenses. (See Chapter 2 for a list of covered hospice services.) You are responsible for the lesser of $5 or 5 percent of the cost of outpatient drugs and 5 percent of the Medicare-approved rate for inpatient respite care. No deductible is required for hospice services.

WHAT MEDICARE WILL NOT PAY FOR

Currently, Medicare will *not* pay for adult day care or adult foster care. It will pay only for respite care for persons who are caring for terminally ill patients. Medicare will pay for nursing care in a life care center only if the regular requirements for home health or skilled nursing-home coverage are met. It will not pay for custodial or intermediate nursing-home care for any length of time, nor will it pay for nursing-home or home-care services on a long-term basis.

WHAT MEDICARE SUPPLEMENT POLICIES PAY FOR

Medicare supplement policies are of little help when it comes to paying for long-term care. These policies are carefully designed to track the services covered by Medicare and pay the deductibles and co-payments due for those services. But if a service isn't covered by Medicare, it usually won't be covered by a Medicare supplement policy.

Some supplement policies cover the co-payment ($74 per day) during the 21st to 100th day in a Medicare-approved skilled nursing home. Keep in mind that if Medicare finds that you do not qualify for skilled nursing-home benefits, most supplement policies will pay nothing.

Some policies are sold to seniors on the understanding that they pay for care in a skilled nursing home after Medicare stops paying on the 100th day. The amounts they pay range from $10 per day to 100 percent of the national average daily charge. Regardless of how much a supplement policy pays for these services, however, the likelihood that you will need skilled nursing care for more than 100 days is small. Before that period ends, most patients are placed in intermediate care or sent home. In either case, virtually all supplement policies will pay nothing.

Medicare supplement policies will not pay for homemaking services, adult day care, respite care, or foster care. A few policies will pay for some short-term, recuperative care at home after a hospital or nursing-home stay. Supplement policies will not pay for custodial care.

WHEN WILL MEDICAID HELP?

Though many people are not poor when they first enter a nursing home, their financial resources soon become depleted as a result of paying for that care. According to one study, after only 13 weeks in a nursing home, nearly half of all elderly people living alone are poor enough for Medicaid. This may be faster than the average time, but nursing-home care can quickly eat up a person's savings. The process of depleting your resources until you qualify for Medicaid is called "spending down."

To qualify for Medicaid, your assets and income must be extremely small. If you are in a nursing home, you must first spend your assets (bank accounts, Individual Retirement Accounts, second homes, stocks, bonds, etc.) down to a few thousand dollars. You are allowed to keep your primary residence, a car, personal clothing, and household items.

If your income is more than a few hundred dollars a month

but less than the cost of nursing-home care, most states allow you to "spend down" this income to qualify for Medicaid. You must contribute all of your income (except for a $30 personal allowance and an allowance for a spouse or other dependent still at home) to your nursing-home expenses. If your income is not enough to pay for all of your nursing-home expenses, Medicaid will pay the portion that you are unable to pay.

Medicaid's eligibility requirements can create serious problems when an elderly person enters a nursing home for an extended period of time and a spouse (frequently, the wife) remains at home without an independent source of income. Medicaid rules could require that nearly all of the couple's assets and income pay for nursing-home expenses, leaving little for the spouse at home to live on. Until recently, often the only way out of this dilemma was divorce.

The Catastrophic Coverage Act of 1988 somewhat improved this situation by requiring that state Medicaid programs total up all of the assets held by either spouse and divide them equally when one spouse enters a nursing home. States must reserve at least $12,000 in assets for the spouse living at home. The law also requires that the spouse who remains at home receive enough of the institutionalized spouse's income to bring her or his income up to about $900 a month. The states can increase these amounts to $60,000 in assets and $1,500 in monthly income. This is one of the few provisions of the Catastrophic Coverage Act that was not repealed in 1989.

If you qualify for Medicaid, the program will pay for skilled nursing-home care and home health care if you need skilled nursing services. Medicaid will also pay for intermediate nursing-home care in almost all states. The services must be provided by nursing homes and home health agencies that meet Medicaid standards and agree to accept Medicaid reimbursement as full payment for their services. Payment is made directly to the provider. Usually, no deductibles or co-payments are required.

While Medicaid usually will not pay for long-term home health care, the federal government has allowed some states to experiment with programs that rely on a variety of home health and community-based services as an alternative to care in nursing homes. The services include:

- rehabilitation services
- respite care
- homemaker services
- adult day care
- foster care
- home-delivered meals
- transportation
- personal care

These programs are still considered experimental and, therefore, are limited to certain geographic areas. (See Chapter 14.)

OTHER PUBLIC PROGRAMS

The Veterans Administration (VA) operates nursing homes, home health programs, adult day-care programs, and hospices that serve eligible veterans. If you are a veteran, you are eligible for VA care if you meet *only one* of the following conditions:

- You are 65 or older.
- You are disabled because of an injury or disease that was incurred or aggravated during active military duty.
- You are retired from active military service because of a disability incurred in the line of duty.
- You are a former prisoner of war.
- You are receiving a VA pension.
- You are eligible for Medicaid.
- You need treatment for a condition related to exposure to Agent Orange or to radiation from nuclear testing while on active duty.

Space in VA facilities and programs is extremely limited. The highest priority is given to veterans who need care for a service-related condition. For more information about care for veterans, contact your local VA office. (Consult the telephone directory under U.S. Government, Veterans Administration.)

THE NEED FOR REFORM

Becoming disabled is a traumatic event, whether it occurs suddenly or gradually. Families are often faced with making agonizing decisions that profoundly affect the lives of individual members. Love, fear, guilt, depression, sorrow, and anger are only some of the emotions that families experience when they confront the problems of long-term disability.

Instead of being a source of comfort and assistance, our current system for paying for long-term care causes hardship and worry. The only practical course open to many disabled people is to deplete their life savings, enter a nursing home, and turn to Medicaid. Because of the high cost of nursing-home care, many disabled people who always had been self-supporting become impoverished in a matter of weeks. Few would maintain that this system is rational, kind, or desirable for any of us.

In the next 30 years, the number of people who will be over 65 is expected to grow from 31 million to 50 million, and the number of people over 85 is expected to double. Already inadequate and expensive, our current system for providing long-term care will be strained even more in the years ahead. Expenses for nursing homes and home care are expected to nearly triple. Under our current system, most of the expenses will be borne by individual families and Medicaid.

This is not the first time our nation has faced a huge economic problem that neither individual efforts nor the commercial marketplace could solve. Our Social Security, unemployment insurance, and Medicare systems were created as solutions to other economic problems in the past. These social insurance programs allow citizens to pool their individual risks by paying into a common fund from which benefits can be drawn in the event of retirement, unemployment, or illness. Benefits are paid as an earned right, not as a public charity.

By extending these principles to long-term care, we can establish a system that is both humane and affordable. Long-term care should be available for all Americans, regardless of age, health, or income. As they now do with Social Security, individuals should contribute to a long-term care fund throughout their working lives. Special rules could ensure that those who are currently near or over 65 receive immediate coverage.

The program should provide comprehensive coverage for home care as well as nursing-home care. Where deductibles and co-payments are necessary, they should be set at levels that won't deny the less affluent fair access to needed care. People could supplement their coverage by buying standardized health insurance policies that pay for deductibles and co-payments.

Establishing this program will not be free. Funds to pay for long-term care will have to be raised through taxes and other means. Overall, these taxes should be based on people's ability to pay. No one welcomes paying taxes, but they are the means by which we collectively buy everything that is considered essential to a civilized society. These include roads, schools, public safety, defense, and health care. Because of the huge cost of long-term care, we cannot protect ourselves against these expenses individually. We can only buy this protection through public means.

IMPROVING MEDICAID

Even if a social insurance program for long-term care is established, we must improve the Medicaid program. Our program for helping poor Americans is often cruel and degrading. Because of inadequate funding, the care is often substandard. We should be disturbed that our medical safety net is in such bad condition. As the problems we now face with long-term care demonstrate, the fall from affluence to poverty can be a swift one, and the people who are forced to turn to Medicaid are often ourselves, our parents, and our children.

Each of these reforms can be achieved. They are workable,

affordable, and like our other social insurance programs, will yield tangible benefits for all Americans for years to come. Of course, none of these programs is perfect, including Social Security, but we are all better off for their existence.

In 1935, it took foresight and strong political leadership to establish Social Security. Now, few politicians would call for shrinking our government or saving taxes by repealing that program. Faced with the challenge of a rapidly aging population, we now need the same courage and foresight to help all of our citizens who need long-term care. Sooner or later, most of us will be among them.

12

Long-term Care Insurance: Should *You* Buy It?

A number of insurance companies sell what they call "nursing home" or "long-term care" insurance. These policies usually pay a set dollar amount for each day that you are in a nursing home. Some policies also pay an amount for home health care. Though buying one of these policies may seem like a good idea, be sure to review them all closely before you decide to buy.

WHO SHOULD AVOID LONG-TERM CARE POLICIES

If your income and assets are low or modest, don't buy a long-term care policy. If it turns out that you need long-term nursing-home care, you probably should look to Medicaid to pay your expenses. For example, if you have an income of $10,000 a year and assets of $10,000 (not including your home), it would not make sense to buy a policy. With nursing homes currently costing about $22,000 a year in most states, you would qualify for Medicaid after about four months as a nursing-home resident. At that point, Medicaid would begin to pay for your nursing-home expenses.

Questions to Ask Before You Buy a Policy

Long-term care insurance is still a relatively new product, and insurance companies are caught between their desire to market them successfully and their fear of incurring huge losses. To guard against such losses, most companies have designed policies with features that minimize their financial risk by reducing the amount of protection given to policyholders. These features include high deductibles, limits on benefits, prior hospitalization or skilled nursing requirements, waiting periods for pre-existing conditions, and reduced coverage for home health and custodial care. In addition, many companies refuse to cover applicants they consider too old or too sick to be profitable to them.

Before you buy a long-term health care policy, ask the following questions:

How much will I have to pay? The premium depends on your age and health. The older you are when you sign up, the more you pay for a policy. For example, if you buy a policy at 55, it might cost you $600 per year. If you first buy a policy when you are 75, the same policy might cost you $3,100 a year. A company also will charge you more if your health is poor.

Long-term care policies are expensive. If you are 65 and in good health, a policy can cost you over $1,100 a year. Paying more does not necessarily mean you're getting a better policy. Some of the policies with the smallest benefits have the biggest price tags.

Once you buy a policy, some companies will increase the premium every few years. Other companies keep the premium the same but reserve the right to raise your premium as long as they do the same for all policyholders in your state. Companies will be tempted to raise rates if expenses for long-term care are more than they expected.

Some companies offer so-called level premiums for life. This means that if the company does decide to raise its rates, your premium will be based on the age you bought the policy, not your current age. This gives you some protection against rate increases, but it does not guarantee you a level premium.

Does the policy provide for a waiver of premium? Some policies will excuse you from paying premiums if you are confined in a nursing home. This feature is called a waiver of premium. It is obviously a desirable feature, for if you need nursing-home services, you may not be in any condition to make the payments. Without a waiver of premium, your policy might lapse just at the time when you need it the most. Pay particular attention to whether the policy you are considering includes this feature and be certain that the policy's language is unambiguous, regardless of the other literature or sales presentation that may accompany it.

Does the policy require that you have received prior hospitalization or a prior level of care before it pays for nursing-home care? Many policies sold before 1989 imposed stiff requirements before they paid any nursing-home benefits. Many required you to be hospitalized for at least three days and that you then entered the nursing home within 10 to 180 days after leaving the hospital. In addition, you had to be staying in the nursing home for the same condition that caused you to be hospitalized. Policies also required that you receive skilled or intermediate nursing care before they would pay for custodial care.

Requirements like these can severely limit the usefulness of a policy. Nearly two-thirds of the patients who enter a nursing home have not been hospitalized beforehand. Conditions such as Alzheimer's disease and arthritis often require nursing-home care without prior hospitalization.

Some states now require that new policies pay nursing-home benefits without requiring prior hospitalization. These states also prohibit new policies from requiring policyholders to have had skilled or intermediate care before they will pay for custodial care. But watch out. These restrictions are still permitted in many states. (See page 000.)

Does the policy set strict requirements for where the nursing-home services need to be provided? All long-term health-care policies specify to some degree where nursing-home services need to be provided, but some are stricter than others. Some policies simply require that a nursing home be licensed by the state before they will pay. Other policies require that a facility meet all of the standards for Medicare certification. Some companies actually spell out detailed staffing and supervision requirements in their policies.

Such strict requirements can prevent you from receiving any benefits, even if you are admitted to a nursing home. In many areas, there is a shortage of nursing-home space, and you may not be able to get into a facility that meets the insurance company's requirements. In that case, the company could refuse to pay your claim. To avoid this problem, look for policies that will pay for stays in any licensed facility.

Will the policy pay for home health services? Policies often contain restrictions on home health care. Some policies cover home health care but only if you would otherwise require care in an institution. Many older policies required that you be confined in a hospital or skilled nursing home before they would pay for home health services. Often, the home health services had to begin within two weeks of leaving the hospital or nursing home. Again, many states are outlawing these kinds of restrictions in new policies, but they are still permitted in some states. (See pages 127–129.)

Will the policy pay for Alzheimer's disease? Some policies are vague about whether they cover Alzheimer's disease. These policies state that they will not pay for care resulting from mental illnesses except those with *demonstrable* organic disease. Alzheimer's disease is definitely an organic disease, but a company facing large claims might insist on tangible proof of the disease. Short of a biopsy or autopsy, that proof may be impossible to produce. If you are unsure whether a policy covers Alzheimer's disease, get a written letter from the company confirming that the condition is covered and that it will accept a letter from your doctor as sufficient proof of its existence.

Also, watch out for policies explicitly stating that they cover Alzheimer's disease but requiring either prior hospitalization or a stay in a skilled nursing home before paying any benefits. Even if Alzheimer's disease is technically covered, these requirements can prevent you from receiving any benefits.

How much will the policy pay per day? The daily benefits paid by long-term care policies vary considerably. Skilled nursing-home benefits range from $25 to more than $100 a day. Some policies pay smaller benefits for intermediate care, custodial care, and home health services. For example, if a policy pays $80 per day for skilled nursing care, it might pay only 75 percent of that for intermediate care, and 50 percent for custodial or home health care.

Will the policy keep up with inflation? Protection against inflation is important, especially if you are buying a policy years before you might need any benefits. In 1977, the average daily charge for care in a skilled nursing home was about $30. By 1985, it had doubled to about $60 a day. If this trend continues, a skilled nursing home will cost an average of $120 a day in 1993.

Some policies do not adjust the amount they pay for inflation. That means if a policy pays $50 a day now, it will still pay only $50 ten years from now, regardless of the cost of nursing-home services. Some companies sell optional riders that raise benefits by a certain percentage each year.

A few companies sell policies that are tied to actual nursing-home costs. As these costs go up, so do the benefits paid by the policy. But be alert. Some companies will limit their risk by promising to pay the "usual and customary" nursing-home charge, but only up to a certain amount per day. If this amount is too low (e.g., $50), the buyer is receiving essentially no protection against inflation.

Inflation protection is expensive. An inflation rider can add between 15 and 40 percent to the cost of a policy. Those policies that pay 100 percent of nursing-home charges can cost two to three times as much as other policies.

How many days and visits will the policy pay for? Some policies pay for an unlimited number of days for each stay in a nursing home, and for an unlimited number of stays. Other policies limit the number of days they cover. For example, a policy might pay for up to 1,095 days (three years) for a single stay, and 1,825 days (five years) for all stays. Some companies use dollar limits instead of specifying a maximum number of days.

Certain policies have lower limits for intermediate and custodial care than for skilled nursing care. Also, policies sometimes limit home health benefits to the same number of days that you received care in a hospital or nursing home.

If you decide to shop for a long-term care policy, it is important to compare these limits closely. Obviously, the best coverage is for an unlimited number of days and stays in a nursing home and no restrictions in the number of home health visits.

When will the policy begin to pay? Does the policy start paying on the first day you go into a nursing home, the 10th day, 20th day, 30th day, or later? This delay in coverage is called the "elimination period." Companies usually let you choose the length of the elimination period; the shorter the period, the more expensive the policy. Before you select a period, ask yourself the following questions:

1. If you went into a nursing home, how long could you afford to pay your own way?

2. Can you afford to pay the added premium for a short elimination period?

3. Would you be better off saving the difference and investing it until you needed to go into a nursing home? (If you didn't need a nursing home, you could use it for other expenses.)

Some policies that cover home health care will pay only after a specified number of visits. If this number is too high, you may be able to collect few, if any, benefits.

What will happen if I'm discharged from a nursing home and need to go back in a relatively short time? Find out what happens if you leave a nursing home and need to be readmitted shortly thereafter. Some policies will start a new elimination period for the second nursing-home stay, during which they will not pay any benefits. Other policies consider all nursing-home stays for the same or related condition within a certain period (for example, six months) the same stay; if you are readmitted during this period, that company will pay benefits for the second stay beginning with the first day.

Can the company cancel the policy? If you buy a long-term care policy, be sure to buy one that is "guaranteed renewable for life." This means that the company cannot cancel you as long as you pay the premium. Some policies are guaranteed renewable, but only up to a certain age (for example, 79). When you reach that specified age, the company can cancel your policy. Some policies offer no protection against cancellation.

Beware of policies that are only "conditionally renewable." These can be canceled if the company decides to cancel all of the policies in the same class. A company might do this if it decided, for example, that too many of its policyholders had reached the age when they would need a lot of long-term care.

Policies sold through groups are not guaranteed renewable. Insurance companies usually reserve the right to cancel the master policy covering the group. If that happens, the group may be able to find another insurance company, or you may be able to convert to an individual policy. In either event, features that are important to you may not exist under the new policy.

What is the loss ratio? If a policy pays out 60 cents in benefits for every dollar consumers pay in premiums, the "loss ratio" is 60 percent. The rest goes to pay for advertising, commissions, company overhead, and profit. Before you buy a policy, ask for the loss ratio. A low loss ratio may indicate that only a few policyholders are receiving benefits from the policy, and/or the benefits paid are extremely small. Long-term care policies should have an expected loss ratio of at least 60 percent.

Does the policy cover pre-existing conditions? Nearly all companies will require you to complete a written questionnaire about your health. The company will ask you to identify any health problems you have experienced in the past six months. Some will go back 12 months, 24 months, five years, or even longer. Generally, companies won't require a physical exam, although some companies may ask your doctor to complete a questionnaire concerning your health.

You should answer all questions about your health accurately and completely. If you forget to include relevant information or you provide inaccurate information, and the company relies on your information, it could later refuse to pay a claim.

Companies use various techniques for limiting their risk for pre-existing conditions. Some companies will cover a pre-existing condition and charge you a higher premium (known as a sub-standard rate). Other companies will impose a waiting period, during which they won't pay for care needed for pre-existing conditions. For example, a policy might not pay for nursing-home stays as a result of pre-existing conditions until six months after you buy the policy. In some states, companies can issue a policy with a "waiver" that excludes coverage for that particular pre-existing condition. Of course, a company could reject you entirely if it believed that you had too many pre-existing conditions to be a good risk for it—for example, if the conditions were likely to land you in a nursing home.

Find out whether there is a waiting period before pre-existing conditions are covered, and how the policy defines pre-existing conditions. In many policies, they are defined as conditions that were diagnosed or treated within six months of the effective date of the policy. Some policies will go back even longer. Waiting periods range from 90 days to two years.

How healthy do I have to be to qualify for the policy? Some companies are more selective than others. Keep in mind that a company may accept you regardless of your health and simply sell you less insurance (by exempting all pre-existing conditions or imposing a long waiting period), or may charge you more (through substandard rates) for the insurance they sell you.

Generally, companies won't accept you if you are over 80 or 85, no matter how healthy you are. If you are younger than that but are certain to need long-term care, you will have difficulty finding a company that will cover you at any price.

What if I decide to drop the policy? If you buy a policy and later decide not to renew it, you may be eligible for a return of some portion of the premiums paid. Be sure to ask the agent or company what you would receive if you decided to cancel the policy.

Will the company be around to pay benefits when I need them? The financial stability of the company from which you buy long-term care insurance is essential to its ability to honor claims in the future. One way to evaluate a company's financial stability is to consult *Best's Insurance Reports*, available in many public libraries. Best's rates insurance companies from A+ (superior) to C (fair) based on a number of factors including their profitability, liquidity, cash reserves, and quality of management. Since you will want a company that will be able to pay claims well into the future, look for policies sold by companies with an A or A+ rating.

BUYING A POLICY

What to Look For in a Policy

Buying long-term care insurance is an expensive proposition. As we noted in the previous section, even if you are willing to spend the money, many policies include restrictions that severely limit their usefulness. In summary, if you are thinking about buying a policy, consider one that

- pays a daily benefit of at least $80
- has an elimination period of not more than 20 days
- has a maximum benefit per stay of at least 1,460 days (four years)
- has an unlimited number of days for all stays
- pays full benefits for skilled, intermediate, and custodial nursing care
- pays nursing-home benefits without requiring a prior hospitalization
- pays home health benefits without
  1. requiring a prior confinement in a hospital or nursing home, or
  2. restricting the number of days of home health care to the number of days of confinement in a hospital or nursing home, or
  3. requiring that you otherwise need care in an institution

- is guaranteed renewable for life
- covers Alzheimer's disease and allows benefits to be paid on the basis of a doctor's certification of the disease
- gives you some protection against rate increases by having a so-called level premium for life
- waives the premium if you are confined to a nursing home
- covers readmission to a nursing home within six months without a new elimination period
- provides protection against inflation in the cost of care
- provides some refund of premiums if you decide to cancel the policy

It may seem cheaper to buy a policy with a level premium when you are 65 or younger. But keep in mind that much of that savings may be eliminated by the additional cost of inflation protection. If you decide to buy a policy without some kind of inflation protection, the benefits will remain level and the value of the policy will be eaten away by inflation.

If you buy a long-term care policy, buy only one. If you already have a long-term care policy, check whether it contains restrictions about prior hospitalization or prior level of care. If it does, ask the company whether you can switch to a policy without these restrictions and still avoid a new waiting period for pre-existing conditions. Also ask whether you can be credited for the premiums you have been paying on your existing policy. Otherwise, the company may charge you higher premiums because you are now several years older and applying for a new policy. If you want higher benefits, ask whether your coverage can be upgraded. If the company refuses, you might decide to apply to another company.

UNFAIR PRACTICES

Many long-term care policies are sold by insurance agents using the same unfair and deceptive practices that they use to sell Medicare supplement policies. If you are buying insurance through an agent, the agent may fill in the application for you and then ask you to sign it. Before you sign an application, make sure that the information in it is accurate and complete. If it isn't, the company could later refuse to pay your claims. You can always mail in an application after inspecting it at your leisure; don't be pressured into signing anything on the spot.

In most states, if an insurance company relies on the information in your application and it subsequently discovers that the information is false or incomplete, the company has the right to rescind your policy and return your premiums. Usually, a company can do this only up to two years after you apply for a policy.

Some companies use this right as a way of getting out of paying claims. Instead of checking your medical history when you submit an application, they will wait until you file a claim. Then such a company will scrutinize your application for any conceivable reason to rescind the policy. This practice is known as post-claims underwriting and it can be highly profitable for an unscrupulous company, since the only policies left after such post-claims cancellations are those without any claims.

Beware of agents who try to get you to lie on an application; they are interested only in making a quick sale, and they actually may be creating a big problem for you in the future. If an agent tries to get you to lie about or cover up a medical condition, insist on telling the truth. If the agent persists, find another one and report the unscrupulous agent to state regulators so that he or she won't cheat others.

You should also be skeptical of companies that promise to cover you quickly (for example, in 24 to 48 hours), or are eager to cover you if you are over 85. Those companies may rely on post-claims underwriting and other unfair practices to avoid paying legitimate claims.

STATE REGULATION OF LONG-TERM CARE INSURANCE

In the past, most states allowed companies to experiment freely with long-term care policies. However, this is changing. As of March 1990, the following states have adopted a "model law" for long-term care policies prepared by the National Association of Insurance Commissioners (NAIC): Arizona, California, Delaware, Florida, Georgia, Hawaii, Idaho, Illinois, Indiana, Iowa, Kansas, Louisiana, Maryland, Montana, Nebraska, Nevada, New Hampshire, New Jersey, New Mexico, North Carolina, North Dakota, Ohio, Oklahoma, Rhode Island, South Carolina, South Dakota, Tennessee, Vermont, Virginia, West Virginia, and Wyoming. The model law

- prohibits policies from covering only skilled nursing care or providing significantly more coverage for skilled care than intermediate or custodial care
- prohibits policies from requiring that home health-care services or prior hospitalization have been provided before paying benefits for a stay in a nursing home
- prohibits companies from going back more than six months in defining pre-existing conditions
- requires that policies cover pre-existing conditions no later than six months after the effective date of the policy
- prohibits policies from excluding Alzheimer's disease
- requires that companies and agents provide consumers with a written outline of coverage at the initial solicitation
- gives consumers the right to return a policy for a full refund within the first 30 days
- requires that policies be guaranteed renewable for life

Despite these protections, the NAIC model law is weak on certain important points. Instead of completely prohibiting prior hospitalization requirements, the law allows states to let insurance companies continue those requirements as long as the companies also offer a policy that doesn't require prior hospitalization before paying benefits. The pitfalls here are obvious.

Companies are still allowed to dig deep into your medical history. While they can't go back more than six months in defining a pre-existing condition, they still can decline your application or charge you more because of conditions you had years ago. In addition, while the model law prohibits companies from canceling your policy because of your age or health, they are still allowed to reject you initially if they decide that your age, health, or medical history makes you an undesirable risk.

A FINAL NOTE ON LONG-TERM CARE INSURANCE

Long-term care policies are still relatively new. Insurance companies are experimenting with various benefits, restrictions, and premium levels. The market is crowded with a number of different policies, and some of the same companies offer two or three in the category. The policies are also changing rapidly. A policy that your neighbor bought two years ago from XYZ Insurance Company may no longer be available today.

Most state regulators have taken a permissive attitude toward long-term care insurance and have stayed out of the way while companies experimented and competed with one another for the health-care dollars of seniors. Because of abuses by companies and agents, some regulators are now trying to catch up with this changing market. Tougher measures have been proposed for the NAIC model code. Even if these measures are adopted, however, they will need to be implemented state by state.

Consequently, people who are interested in purchasing long-term care insurance should take the time to examine these policies carefully and decide for themselves whether the protection they offer is worth the price. Meanwhile, all of us should urge our state insurance commissions to adopt the reforms needed to correct the abuses of the insurance industry before waiting for the NAIC to act.

13

Are You Ready?

Whether it's at age 62, 65, or later, retirement usually means some important changes in your health insurance. The steps outlined in this chapter will help to ensure that those changes occur smoothly. You should take certain steps well before you retire, while others can be postponed until you are closer to retirement.

CHECK YOUR EXISTING COVERAGE

Before you retire, spend some time carefully checking your existing coverage. If you are covered by your employer's group health insurance plan, find out if you are entitled to any coverage after you retire. Your employer or union representative should be able to tell you

- whether the group plan covers retirees
- what services are covered
- whether there are any premiums, deductibles, and/or co-payments you will be responsible for
- whether the group plan covers spouses
- how the plan works with Medicare

If you are not covered by a group plan and have an individual policy, call the insurance company and find out what will happen to your coverage when you qualify for Medicare. Many policies will automatically convert to a Medicare supplement policy when you reach your 65th birthday.

AVOID ANY BREAKS IN COVERAGE

If you or your spouse will be under 65 when you retire, take special care to ensure that you will have continuous coverage after you retire. Keep in mind that Medicare will not pay for your health-care expenses until you reach age 65. The same is true for your spouse.

For example, if you retire before age 65 and your employer's plan does not cover retirees, you will be facing a break in coverage from the time your retire to when you reach 65. If your spouse is also under 65, currently covered by your employer group plan, and not eligible for any other group plan, there will also be a break in his or her coverage until age 65.

If it appears that retirement will mean a break in coverage, investigate the following solutions:

Continuing Your Group Coverage

If you are covered by an employer group plan, you may have the right to continue your group coverage at your own expense for up to 18 months. Generally, the premium you will have to pay will be substantially less than the cost of buying an individual policy. Also, you won't have to worry about qualifying for a new policy or having to undergo a waiting period for pre-existing conditions. At the end of 18 months, you may have the right to convert to an individual policy. (See the next paragraph for further details.) To find out whether you have a right to continue or convert your group coverage, contact your employer or union representative. These rights usually extend to a spouse who has been covered by group plans.

Converting Your Group Coverage

If you are covered by an employer group plan, you may have the right to convert your group coverage to an individual policy.

Conversion policies are often expensive, however, and because of this, you should compare the conversion policy offered you to policies offered by other companies. The advantage of conversion is that the company that has covered you must issue you a conversion policy regardless of your health, and no waiting period is required for pre-existing conditions.

Keeping an Individual Policy

If you and your spouse are covered by an individual policy, you may need to keep that policy until both of you are over 65, and then shop for a Medicare supplement policy. (Medicare supplement policies should not be confused with long-term care policies.) This is particularly true if either of you is in poor health or has a medical condition that requires ongoing treatment. Strict health requirements and waiting periods for pre-existing conditions may make it impractical to shop for a new policy before you qualify for Medicare.

Check with Social Security

Before you retire, check with the Social Security Administration to see whether you have enough work credits to qualify for Social Security retirement benefits and Medicare. The first step in this process is to call your local Social Security office and ask for a Request for Social Security Statement of Earnings. (Consult your telephone directory under U.S. Government, Social Security Administration.) When you get the form, fill it out, double-check your Social Security number to make sure it's correct, and mail the request to your Social Security office.

Several weeks later, you should receive a Summary Statement of Earnings. When you get this summary, call or drop by your Social Security office. Using the information from the summary, a case worker can tell you whether you qualify for Social Security retirement benefits, and if so, approximately how much you can expect to receive. The case worker also should be able to estimate how much more you would receive if you delay applying for benefits. This information could affect your decision about whether to retire at 62, 65, or later. If you qualify for Social Security retirement benefits, you will also qualify for Medicare when you reach 65.

FIND DOCTORS WHO WILL ACCEPT MEDICARE ASSIGNMENT

For the reasons described in Chapter 2, choosing a doctor who accepts Medicare assignment can save you a lot of money. By starting early, it will be easier to discuss this topic with your current doctors, and if necessary, to find ones who will agree to limit their charges to the Medicare-approved amount.

Before you retire, find out whether your doctor(s) accepts Medicare assignment. The best way is to call the doctor's office and explain that you would like the doctor to accept assignment for all services once you qualify for Medicare.

If your doctor refuses to accept assignment, consider finding another doctor. The *Medicare Participating Physician/Supplier Directory* lists all of the doctors in your area who have agreed to accept Medicare assignment for all of the services provided to persons covered by Medicare. Copies are available from the insurance company that handles your Medicare claims. (See Appendix A.)

SIGN UP FOR MEDICARE

Three months before you retire, sign up for your Social Security retirement benefits. You can get the necessary form from your local Social Security office. By signing up for Social Security, you will also be signing up for Medicare. Your Medicare coverage will begin on the first day of the month that you turn 65.

If you don't want to begin receiving your Social Security retirement benefits until after 65, but you want your Medicare coverage to begin at 65, you need to fill out Form HCFA 18-F5 at your local Social Security office. That form simply lets the government know that you would like your Medicare coverage to start.

GET TO KNOW THE
RESOURCES IN YOUR COMMUNITY

In most communities, there are a number of agencies and programs that provide information and assistance to senior citizens. Some communities offer insurance counseling programs that can help answer questions about Medicare, unravel the complexities of private insurance, and alert you to unfair practices that are prevalent in your community. There are also programs that can provide you with legal assistance if you run into problems with Medicare, Medicaid, hospitals, nursing homes, doctors, or other health-care providers.

Get to know these resources. Once you do, you will be better prepared to deal with any problems that occur, and you will be able to help others who may be struggling to solve a problem. (For the agencies in your area, consult your telephone directory under U.S. or state government listings (Elderly Assistance or Senior Citizens Assistance), or the Yellow Pages listings (Senior Citizens' Service Organizations or Social Service Organizations). (See Appendix B.)

ORGANIZE YOUR PAPERS

Take a couple of hours to set up a system for organizing your papers. An organized system will make it easier for you to find important information and to keep track of your bills. We suggest that you organize your papers by using five file folders, as follows:

1. **Insurance identification cards.** Keep copies of your Medicare card and other insurance identification cards in this folder. The originals should be kept in your wallet. If you lose the originals, you can use the identification numbers on the copies to submit claims and order replacement cards.

2. **Insurance policies.** If you have a Medicare supplement policy, a long-term care policy, and/or other private insurance pol-

icies, keep them in this folder. For each policy, write down on the inside cover of the folder

- the name of the policy
- the policy number
- when premiums are due (for example, annually, quarterly, monthly, etc.)

This information is important. If you have an accident or illness and you can't talk, a relative or friend can quickly find out what policies you have and pay the premiums on time to keep those policies in effect.

3. Claim-tracking form. Keep track of your Medicare and other insurance claims by using a tracking form. (For a sample form, see Appendix C.) Write down when you submitted a claim and when it was paid. Keep the form in this folder and use it to see whether a claim has been submitted, is still outstanding, or has been paid.

4. Bills to be submitted. Put all the bills that you need to submit claims for in this folder. When you submit a claim, transfer the bill (or bills) to the Outstanding Claims file.

5. Outstanding claims. Keep copies of all claims that you have submitted to Medicare or your private insurance company in this folder until the claim has been paid.

6. Completed claims. When a claim is paid, transfer it from the Outstanding Claims folder to the Completed Claims folder. Attach any explanation you receive from Medicare or your insurance company about the claim.

7. Extra claim forms. Keep extra claim forms in this folder so they are readily available when you need to make a claim.

WHERE TO KEEP YOUR PAPERS

Keep your papers where you can easily get them. A file drawer or a large cardboard box at home will do fine. Don't put your insurance policies in a safety-deposit box. These papers are of value only to you, and no one is likely to steal them. If your policies are locked in a safe-deposit box and you have a medical emergency, your family may never know that you have these policies, and might allow them to lapse.

Be sure your spouse knows where your papers are (and that you briefly explain how they are organized) in case you become incapacitated. If you live alone, show a close relative or friend where they are. If you move the papers, be sure to tell your spouse, relative, or friend about the new location.

A RETIREMENT TIME LINE

There is no magic formula for getting ready for retirement. Generally, the earlier you start, the easier it will be. By gathering the information you need early, you can explore alternatives and adjust your plans where necessary. For this reason, we suggest the following timetable:

24 months before retirement: Check on your existing health insurance coverage and with Social Security.

12 months before retirement: Check with your doctors regarding Medicare assignment and find out about local information resources.

3 months to retirement: Sign up for Social Security retirement benefits.

1 month to retirement: Set up your filing system and let others know where you will keep your papers.

The transition from work to retirement is one of the biggest changes in your life. Don't rush. Give yourself the time you need to gather the necessary information to make sound decisions.

14

What You Can Do to Make the System Work Better

Throughout this book, we have described some of the problems facing older Americans on Medicare. These problems include not enough doctors who accept Medicare assignment, abusive practices by insurance companies and agents, and a general lack of government support for long-term care. In many communities, citizens have joined together to begin to address these and other problems. Some of these efforts involve education while others seek to change the way doctors, hospitals, insurance companies, and government programs treat older people. The following are some of the ways local organizations are working to improve the system.

CONTROLLING THE COST OF DOCTORS' SERVICES

Most doctors still refuse to accept assignment for all of their Medicare-eligible patients. This means that they are free to charge patients more than the Medicare-approved rate. The likelihood of finding a doctor who accepts assignment varies from state to state, and even from community to community. As of January 1989, Alabama had the highest percentage of doctors who agreed to accept assignment for all their Medicare-eligible patients (75.9 percent), and Idaho had the lowest (16.0 percent).

Nationwide, the percentage was 40.7 percent. (For information about your state, consult the table in Appendix D.)

In many communities, senior groups have conducted successful campaigns to increase the number of doctors who accept Medicare assignment. Depending on the objectives and resources of the particular group, these campaigns have targeted local medical societies, hospitals, and doctors. In a few cases, statewide campaigns have led to legislation prohibiting doctors from charging patients more than the Medicare-approved amount. Remember that doctors and other health-care providers profit from patients whose fees are partially or fully reimbursed by Medicare dollars. Losing numbers of patients would be costly indeed to them and the health-care facilities with which they are affiliated. The following are examples of how some communities have begun to control the cost of doctors' services:

Harrisburg, Pennsylvania

The Dauphin County Council of Senior Citizens in Harrisburg, Pennsylvania, conducted an intensive campaign to persuade local doctors to accept Medicare assignment. One of its first steps was to compile a directory of local physicians, showing their specialty and the percentage of cases they took on assignment. Good grades were given to doctors with high assignment rates, and poor grades were given to those with low rates.

When the local medical association refused to negotiate with the council, its members wrote directly to 248 physicians and asked each to agree to accept Medicare assignment. The letter promised that doctors who agreed would be listed in a new directory that would be available through the 54 organizations that had endorsed the campaign. The council's campaign and the intense media coverage that accompanied it resulted in a 63 percent increase in the number of local doctors accepting assignment.

Cape Cod, Massachusetts

Prior to enactment of a state law prohibiting excess charges, a coalition of organizations in Cape Cod, Massachusetts, including

Cape United Elderly, secured agreements from two community hospitals requiring all physicians with admitting privileges to accept Medicare assignment and Medicaid patients. In addition to educating the media about the lack of affordable medical services on Cape Cod, the group organized mass demonstrations to focus public attention on local hospitals and physicians.

Montana

The Montana Senior Citizens Association negotiated an agreement with eight hospitals throughout the state requiring each of these hospitals to waive all or part of the Medicare hospital deductible, and hospital doctors to limit their fees to the Medicare-approved amount. The hospitals also agreed to provide free transportation to and from the hospital or doctor's office, offer preventive health seminars, and help patients with their insurance claims.

Champaign, Illinois

The Champaign County Health Care Consumers in Champaign, Illinois, negotiated an agreement requiring a local hospital to waive the Medicare deductible for inpatient hospital care and the 20 percent co-payment for doctors' services for low-income seniors. The hospital agreed to give other seniors a 25 to 35 percent discount for covered services.

The group was successful, in part, because it was able to convince the hospital representatives that reducing the cost of health-care services was good for business. From its research, it knew that the hospital was facing financial problems. The group was able to demonstrate that by reducing the cost of services to Medicare recipients, the hospital would be able to attract more patients.

State Legislation

Citizen activism has resulted in four states passing legislation that prohibits doctors from charging seniors more than the Medicare-approved amount for covered services. In Connecticut and Massachusetts, doctors are prohibited from imposing any charges on Medicare patients in excess of Medicare-approved amounts. In Vermont and Rhode Island, state law prohibits doctors from imposing such excess charges on low-income seniors.

In some states, powerful state medical associations have been able to defeat proposed legislation. But even when these bills are defeated, they help to educate the legislature, the media, and the public about the problem of escalating doctors' fees.

IMPROVING MEDICARE SUPPLEMENT POLICIES

In most states, dozens of different Medicare supplement policies are on the market. Some of the differences among the policies are important, but many are trivial. The lack of standardization makes it easier for unscrupulous agents to sell policies based on misrepresentation and confusion instead of meeting a genuine need for supplemental protection.

In Massachusetts, a state law standardizes Medicare supplement policies into one of three coverage groups: high, medium, and low. The coverage for each group of policies is specified by the law, making it easier for buyers to compare policies. In addition, the state reviews the premiums charged for Medicare supplement policies to prevent insurance companies from gouging the elderly.

The standardization of policies and the regulation of rates have increased the benefits paid to buyers in Massachusetts. A report by the General Accounting Office found that policies in Massachusetts returned 98 cents in benefits for each dollar paid in premiums, compared to the average of 60 cents for other Medicare supplement policies. Over objections from the insurance industry, California, Wisconsin, and Minnesota have also passed laws requiring the standardization of Medicare supplement policies.

WAKING UP THE STATE WATCHDOGS

In many states, insurance commissioners are more like sleeping hounds than vigilant watchdogs. As a result, insurance companies and their agents freely engage in a wide range of unfair and deceptive practices aimed at elderly consumers. In several states, senior organizations and consumer groups have prodded commissioners to assume a more active role in protecting the elderly against unscrupulous companies and agents.

In California, a coalition of seniors and consumer organizations led by Consumers Union forced that state's commissioner to crack down on phony insurance company mailings to senior citizens. When the commissioner refused to take other actions needed to police the insurance industry, the groups convinced the state legislature to pass laws requiring that the commissioner publish a guide to long-term care insurance, establish a toll-free hotline for consumer complaints, and standardize Medicare supplement policies.

A few state commissioners have gone further in protecting the elderly. In Washington State, the commissioner has published a guide that provides side-by-side comparisons of the Medicare supplement policies sold in that state and has been among the leaders in regulating long-term care insurance to make certain that needed coverage is provided at fair rates.

OPPOSING EXCESSIVE INSURANCE RATES

In many states, insurance companies must apply to the state's insurance commissioner before they can raise their rates. Because the public is almost always unaware that the company is seeking an increase, there is usually no opposition.

In Rhode Island, the Coalition for Consumer Justice defeated a proposed increase in the cost of Medicare supplement policies sold by Blue Cross. Blue Cross claimed that it needed an increase because of rising doctors' fees. The coalition showed that, in fact, Congress had frozen doctors' fees for the period in question.

In addition to opposing proposed rate hikes, groups of consumers can push for the requiring of increased public participation in the rate-setting process. This can be achieved through laws that require advance notice to the public of rate-hike applications and give consumer representatives a fair opportunity to examine the companies' rate request, cross-examine company representatives, and present their own testimony and evidence. In California, insurance companies are required to pay for the attorneys and expert witnesses that consumers need to oppose higher rates.

PROVIDING LOCAL ASSISTANCE FOR SENIORS

Recognizing the need for special assistance, some states have established health-insurance counseling programs that provide advice and information to seniors, often on a one-to-one basis. These programs currently operate in California, Idaho, Indiana, Iowa, Maryland, Massachusetts, New Jersey, New Mexico, North Carolina, Ohio, and Washington State. (See Appendix C.)

The programs are staffed by volunteer counselors who are trained and supervised by staff experts. The counselors provide general information about Medicare and private insurance, help seniors make decisions about buying insurance, resolve individual problems, and help to uncover abuses. These counseling programs can also provide important information to legislative bodies and regulatory agencies concerning the problems seniors experience with Medicare and private insurance.

IDENTIFYING AND EXAMINING
LOCAL NURSING-HOME RESOURCES

When it comes to finding and evaluating nursing-home services, many families have little to go on other than their own instincts and efforts. Some groups are trying to address this problem by researching local nursing homes and publishing the results in a directory.

In Seattle, Washington, the nonprofit Washington Nursing Home Rating Service publishes two guides that evaluate 120 nursing homes in a five-county area. The guides describe the facilities, admission policy, staff qualifications, and cost of each nursing home. In addition, they identify the problems uncovered by state inspectors and indicate whether these problems have been corrected. In the District of Columbia, the National Council of Senior Citizens has published a consumer guide to nursing homes in the D.C. area.

When carefully researched and clearly presented, publications like these can be an immediate help to the families of people who need long-term care. The research can also uncover problems in the availability, delivery, and cost of nursing-home services and lead to changes in the nursing-home industry.

DEFENDING THE MEDICAID PROGRAM

Middle-class seniors often believe that with Medicare, they will never have to depend on the Medicaid program, which they perceive as reserved for the very poor.

But many older people must look to their state Medicaid program for financial help, and many middle-class seniors eventually are forced to do so if their own resources become depleted by long-term disability.

In many states, Medicaid programs are routinely targeted for budget cuts. This means reducing the number of people who are eligible for the program, cutting benefits, or both. Across the country, coalitions representing the poor, the disabled, women, children, and the elderly have fought to prevent further cuts in Medicaid. Through detailed research and creative presentations, they have demonstrated to state legislators that proposed cuts are unnecessary, counterproductive, and cruel. Where budget cuts were unavoidable, the coalitions often have identified different ways to reduce spending without harming Medicaid recipients.

Defending state Medicaid programs is among the most important challenges facing the elderly. If these programs are not adequately funded, it will mean even more hardship for low-income seniors. By joining with other groups that rely on Medicaid, you will be able to make the strongest case for a fair and just level of funding.

IMPROVING MEDICAID

State Medicaid programs can be improved in two ways. They can be expanded to include seniors who are poor but above the official poverty line, and the services covered by Medicaid can be expanded to include a range of home health and community-based services.

Helping the Medically Needy

Unless special measures are implemented, older people whose incomes are slightly above the poverty line receive no help from Medicaid, no matter how sick they get or how much they need to spend on medical care. By law, states have the option of expanding Medicaid to include these and other "medically needy" people. Thirty-five states have expanded coverage, but 15 have not. The states that do not cover the medically needy are Alabama, Alaska, Arizona, Colorado, Delaware, Idaho, Indiana, Mississippi, Missouri, Nevada, New Mexico, Ohio, South Carolina, South Dakota, Wyoming, and the U.S. island possession of Guam.

In Oregon, Iowa, and Rhode Island, broad coalitions representing the poor, the disabled, mothers, children, and the elderly have convinced governors and state legislatures to include a "medically needy" category in their Medicaid program. Coalitions such as these can improve the lives of low-income people of all ages.

Home Care and Community-Based Services

Normally, state Medicaid programs can pay only for nursing-home care and for extremely limited home health care. A state can ask the federal government to waive certain provisions of the Medicaid Act to allow the state to pay for home health and community-based services for people who would otherwise need to be institutionalized. This process is known as "applying for a waiver."

Under the waiver process, states may target a number of groups, such as the elderly, the physically disabled, the mentally retarded, and the mentally ill for home and community-based services as an alternative to institutional care. States may select specific geographic areas, such as a city, county, or region, where home health and community-based services may be provided.

The alternative services could include case management, homemaker services, home health services, personal care, adult day care and foster care, transportation, meal services, respite care, emergency response systems, and other services that would help people remain in the community. The Health Care Financing Administration periodically publishes a "Medicaid Waiver Fact Sheet" that summarizes the waivers granted for home and community-based services for each state. To get a copy, write to: Office of Publications, Health Care Financing Administration, 6325 Security Boulevard, Baltimore, MD 21207. The fact sheet will give you an idea of the types of alternative services your state and other states are applying for. To qualify for a waiver, states must show that the new services will not exceed the cost of comparable institutional care.

Local organizations that are concerned about the lack of home health and community-based services can play an important role by persuading state officials to seek a waiver. By carefully researching and documenting the lack of services and the hardship imposed on local families, you can put together a powerful case for seeking additional services.

Initially, state officials may be reluctant to apply for a waiver. The waiver process is still relatively new, and there are a number of technical rules that officials must follow. In addition, local nursing homes are likely to oppose a waiver, since more home health and community-based services will mean fewer nursing-home patients. To overcome this resistance, you may need to enlist the support of local officials and the media. Both can help to ensure that state officials follow through and obtain the necessary waiver.

PREVENTING INCOME DISCRIMINATION

Under our current system, there are basically four sources of money to pay for health care: private funds, private insurance, Medicare, and Medicaid. When federal and state budgets are constrained, limits are often placed on the amount that Medicare and Medicaid will pay for covered services. If these limits are lower than those paid by private individuals or by private insurance, doctors and other health-care providers have an incentive either to turn away Medicare and Medicaid patients or to reduce the care they provide to them. As the gap widens, more hospitals, nursing homes, and doctors will care for patients only if they have expensive private insurance, or can pay their own expenses from private funds.

Several states are attempting to address this problem by establishing a uniform rate regardless of the source of payment. Maryland, Massachusetts, New York, and New Jersey have established a system for getting uniform hospital rates. In Minnesota, nursing homes are prohibited from charging their private-pay patients more than the state Medicaid reimbursement rate. Rate-setting systems such as these must be carefully designed to ensure that all patients, regardless of income, have access to quality care.

SUPPORTING NATIONAL REFORMS

Some reforms, such as expanding Medicare to cover long-term care, can only be implemented at the national level. When coordinated with federal efforts in Washington, state and local organizations can play a crucial role by showing elected officials that people in their state or district need these reforms.

In New Jersey, for example, the Home Health Agency Assembly, along with several community groups, convinced one of their senators to hold local hearings on the need for long-term care. Some of the most moving testimony came from homebound patients and their families who made their comments on videotape, since they could not appear in person.

Hearings such as these can help to persuade politicians who

are opposed to government assistance for long-term care (and those who are undecided) that they should support such assistance for political as well as humane reasons.

CONDUCTING A SUCCESSFUL CAMPAIGN

Some of these reforms are easier to achieve than others, but they all require a substantial amount of work. In many cases, it takes the knowledge, experience, talent, and influence of more than one group to bring about the desired change. Here are some important steps to take when you join with others in pressing for the types of reforms described in this chapter.

1. Learn from people who have undertaken similar campaigns. Chances are that the problems you are experiencing in your community also exist in other areas. If you are just starting out, it's worthwhile to contact people and organizations who have attempted to address similar problems in their community. In many cases, they will be able to give you valuable information about how to research and document problems, solutions that might work, where to look for potential allies, how to overcome opposition, and pitfalls to avoid. They also might be willing to share survey forms, reports, news releases, fact sheets, videotapes, and other materials they used in their campaign.

A good place to start is Families, U.S.A., which publishes *The Best Medicine: Organizing Local Health Care Campaigns*, a guide for people and organizations interested in reforming the health-care system. You can contact Families, U.S.A., at 1334 G Street N.W., Washington, D.C., 20005, 202-737-6340. Families, U.S.A., also funds a wide range of efforts aimed at bringing about fundamental changes in instituutions and attitudes affecting the elderly. Many of the projects described in this chapter received funding or technical support from Families, U.S.A.

2. Research problems thoroughly and accurately. All successful campaigns are based on thorough research. The research may involve identifying the nursing homes in your area and compiling the results of state inspections. It may involve conducting a survey of local doctors to see whether they will accept Medicare assignment or treat patients who are on Medicaid. In many cases, it will involve asking your members what they think about the local health-care system, and documenting the problems they have in receiving needed care.

The main purpose of such research is to understand exactly what the problems are so that effective solutions can be developed. The facts you uncover are also needed to convince decision makers that the problems you have identified should be addressed.

Whatever problem you are confronting, make sure that your research is both accurate and thorough. Your work will be scrutinized by decision makers, the media, and your opponents. Superficial research could end your campaign and damage your group's credibility. Solid research will withstand attack and earn your group a reputation for backing your proposals with hard evidence.

3. Develop solutions that will work in your community. Once you've identified the problem, give a lot of thought to possible solutions. Situations that seem simple often have some hidden twists. The problems may require a more complex solution than you first envisioned.

Be sure that the solution you are considering will work in your community. The fact that a particular approach has succeeded in one community does not guarantee that it will work in yours. For example, requiring all doctors to accept Medicare assignment may be counterproductive in a community where there are too few doctors, or where the Medicare-approved rate of reimbursement is unrealistically low. In this situation, such a previously successful solution might backfire, and instead of charging seniors less, doctors may simply refuse to accept them as patients.

Before you commit yourself to one solution, consult with experts who are sympathetic to your cause. They might confirm that you are on target, in which case you can proceed with confidence, or they might suggest other approaches to solving the problem. Be open to their experience, and profit by their advice.

4. Enlist the support of other groups. Many of the important reforms described in this chapter were achieved because groups representing the elderly joined with those representing the poor, disabled, women, children, and consumers. By forming coalitions like the Mississippi Coalition for Mothers and Babies, the Coalition for Consumer Justice, and the Cape Cod Health Care Coalition, groups were able to achieve results far beyond those that would have been accessible had they worked alone.

Forming a coalition is often essential to fighting the usually powerful forces that will oppose any change. The opposition may come from nursing homes that would like to control the information available to consumers, from doctors who would like to impose higher charges on their patients, or from insurance companies and agents who would like to continue to sell seniors policies that they don't need. A coalition can help to overcome such opposition by demonstrating broad public support for your reforms.

5. Identify and assess your opponents. Take some time to identify who will oppose you, and learn as much as you can about them. For example, if you expect opposition from the local medical association, find out who the association represents, whether there are dissident groups that have broken away from the association, the arguments and tactics the association is likely to use, who leads the association, their reputation in the community, and whom they respect and listen to. All of this information will help you in planning your campaign.

If the opposition seems overwhelming, explore ways to reduce the amount of opposition and still achieve something important. For example, if you are proposing uniform rates for both hospitals *and* nursing homes, you assure yourself fierce opposition from both the hospital and nursing-home lobbies. By limiting your proposal to only hospitals, you may reduce your opposition considerably. If you are successful, you can propose a similar system for nursing homes, and point to the hospital legislation you have won as a model for it.

6. Decide on your overall goal and how you will get there.
Before you launch your campaign, make sure you know what
you are trying to achieve. Before you begin, write down the overall goal of your group or coalition. Setting a broad goal is usually
desirable, because it will help to keep the group or coalition working together after the initial campaign. For example:

> Our coalition's objective is to ensure that people can get the
> medical care they need regardless of their age or wealth. Of
> particular concern to our coalition are the unmet needs of
> the elderly, people with low incomes, children, the disabled,
> and those people who are uninsured.

Next, write down how the effort you are planning will further
your overall objectives, for example:

> If successful, our campaign to expand the Medicaid program
> to cover the medically needy will provide more medical care
> to all of these groups.

Then write down some intermediate goals for your campaign.
If you are trying to bring about a big change, you might not
reach your ultimate goal right away. These intermediate goals
will help to keep you on track. For example:

> Because extending Medicaid to the medically needy will re-
> quire a substantial increase in the Medicaid budget, it is im-
> portant that the coalition take the time to thoroughly educate
> the public, the media, the legislature, and the governor about
> the problem. Our intermediate goals for the campaign should
> be:
>
> **Year 1** • Official commission established to investigate the
> medical needs of low-income people
> • Commission to include several coalition members
> and to hold statewide hearings to learn directly
> from low-income people
> • Widespread media coverage of hearings followed
> by placing editorials calling on state officials to ad-
> dress the problem

- Report on findings of the commission, etc.
Year 2 • Legislation introduced to extend Medicaid to those who are defined as medically needy
- Hearings held by both houses of the state legislature
- Legislation approved by one house
- Extensive media coverage and editorial support
Year 3 • Legislation approved by both houses
- Legislation signed by the governor
- Agency with responsibility for administration and enforcement begins to implement the new law
- More media coverage and editorial support

Be sure to consult the other members of your coalition about what the goals should be, and to get their agreement before you proceed. Use what you've written down to plan your campaign and also to mark your progress.

7. Be alert if you are offered a compromise. One of the most difficult decisions that will face a coalition is when to compromise. As your efforts become effective, you may be offered a small step toward your proposed solution. For example, if you are seeking mandatory Medicare assignment for all doctors, you might be offered instead a commission to study escalating doctors' fees.

Usually, there are no clear-cut answers when a compromise is offered. Of course, no one would compromise if winning were a sure thing. The problem is that, most of the time, you won't know whether you will win or lose, or what form that win or loss will take. There is also the possibility that while you may lose this time, you might win eventually.

Because of these uncertainties, decisions about when to compromise require some careful political judgment combined with a keen sensitivity to the principles that underlie a group or coalition. Without both, you may miss valuable opportunities to advance your cause, or you may forsake the overall objectives you are trying to achieve.

Before accepting or rejecting a compromise, consult with the other members of your coalition. They may see problems or possibilities that you missed. In any case, you will need their support.

One way to assess a proposed compromise is whether it prevents (or delays) the coalition from achieving its objectives, or whether it makes achieving those objectives lmore likely. For example, you might reject a proposed study commission if the commission will (a) create the public impression that the problem was solved, (b) be stacked against you, or (c) take years to study the problem. Conversely, you might accept the compromise if (a) the views of your coalition will be adequately represented on the commission, (b) the commission will have a chance to hear firsthand from the people you are trying to help, (c) one of the commission's duties will be to present a comprehensive plan to address the problems you have identified, or (d) the commission will have a stature and a credibility that will be hard for decision makers to ignore. Making this assessment will be easier if your group or coalition has clearly identified its overall goal as well as what it considers are acceptable intermediate steps toward those objectives.

8. Try to keep the coalition united. When faced with a broad coalition armed with unassailable facts, your opponents may propose measures that will help one group at the expense of another, seeking to divide and conquer. For example, state officials may offer to expand services for the elderly on the condition that these services be paid for by cuts in services to the poor.

Don't fall victim to these tactics. When a coalition is split, all of the groups in it are weakened, making it less likely that you will be able to secure other reforms or protect your gains from future attack. Also, by fighting among one another, you will be made to appear selfish, willing to sacrifice the needs of others, and without any moral basis for your proposal. Again, it is easier to keep a coalition united if the groups have agreed in advance what their overall goal is and how they will go about achieving that goal. That way, your coalition will avoid being co-opted by opponents who seek to weaken its strength as a unit.

9. Remember that there are no permanent victories, nor any permanent defeats. Even if your efforts result in a stunning victory, be aware that those hard-fought reforms could vanish unless you are vigilant. Your opponents will be seeking ways to repeal those reforms in a subsequent session of the legislature, overturn them in court, or water them down at the regulatory level. Be prepared for these efforts and if necessary, fight to preserve your victory.

In the same way, keep in mind that no defeat is permanent. By raising the issue, you have educated decision makers, the media, and the public about the problem, and developed your organizing skills. It may take more research, more organizing, and more education, but, if the problem is a serious one, eventually those in charge will need to find a solution. Like your opponents, you should never give up.

THE FUTURE OF MEDICARE

Medicare will need to undergo substantial reform to keep up with our aging population. As Americans live longer and have smaller families, both the number and the proportion of older people will increase substantially. The Census Bureau estimates that over the next 50 years, the elderly population will grow twice as fast as the population under 65. Because of medical advances, persons over 85 will be the fastest-growing segment of the elderly population.

As the number and the age of Medicare beneficiaries increase, the cost of the Medicare program (already approaching 10 percent of the federal budget) will increase dramatically. The Congressional Budget Office estimates that the cost of the Medicare program is expected to increase by 15 percent a year. The need for long-term care will also increase.

At the same time, fewer younger Americans means fewer workers to pay for each senior receiving Medicare benefits. Currently, there are about four workers contributing to Medicare for each Medicare beneficiary. By the middle of the 21st century, only about two workers will be supporting each beneficiary.

These trends are serious enough to bankrupt the Medicare program. The board of trustees that oversees the Hospital Insurance Trust Fund (Part A) has estimated that the fund could be insolvent as early as 1999. The smaller Supplemental Medical Insurance Trust Fund (Part B) is experiencing similar escalation in costs and is kept afloat only through higher Part-B premiums and larger subsidies from the federal budget.

As our recent experience with catastrophic care legislation illustrates, Americans are deeply ambivalent about health care. We demand programs that will improve our health, yet we are often unwilling to consider higher taxes to pay for them. We call for far-reaching improvements in our health system, yet many of us are outraged when we are asked to pay for those improvements.

Until now, older Americans have been able to escape this contradiction by calling for new programs and asking that working-age citizens pay for most of the costs. It is doubtful whether this approach can continue to work in the near future. As the ratio of workers to Medicare beneficiaries decreases, we will reach a practical limit to how much we can ask workers to contribute to Medicare. At some point, the burden on workers becomes crushing.

Nor can we ignore the pressing health needs of younger Americans. There are 37 million men, women, and children in this country who have no health insurance. By contrast, only about 300,000 people over 65 lack health insurance. For these uninsured Americans, even basic health care is unaffordable, and every illness is a crisis.

Other social needs also demand our urgent attention. Adults who have poor health, poor housing, and poor education will make poor workers. In desperate need themselves, they will be in no position to contribute to the health and welfare of others. We need to address these problems at the same time that we find solutions to the problems in Medicare.

The crisis brewing in the Medicare program makes it imperative that we reassess what we want from our health-care system and what we are willing to pay. Our current system has resulted in longer lives and better health for many. But it has also led to more lives that are severely limited by chronic conditions requiring long-term care. Our system also creates vastly inequitable levels of care. While expensive, high-technology cures are available to some, many Americans are denied access to even basic care. Finally, our current system is unaffordable. Its costs are overwhelming both our individual and governmental budgets.

As a nation, we will need to strike a balance between acute care and long-term care, between advanced medicine and basic health needs, between health care for the elderly and other social programs. This will not be easy. At the heart of this debate will be moral questions such as: How long do we need to live? How much pain should we be ready to endure? How much disability can we survive? What obligations do the young have to the old? What obligations do the old owe to the young? What is the relationship between health and individual happiness, between health and the common good? Questions like these are not amenable to technical solutions. Nor are they best resolved through a single-minded pursuit of one's own self-interest in the political process.

Older Americans have a large stake in this debate—not just as individual patients who may need care and as individual taxpayers who may be asked to pay for it—but also as citizens interested in the overall health and well-being of our nation. They will play a crucial and, at times, a decisive role in resolving the difficult problems facing us. As a group, older Americans can choose to focus their considerable political power solely on preserving and enhancing their own security. Or they can use this power to place our health-care system into proper balance and improve the security of all Americans.

Appendix A:
Insurance Companies That Process Medicare Claims

The following companies have been hired as carriers by Medicare to handle Part-B (Medical Insurance) claims. The Medicare Insurance carrier serving your area can provide you with claim forms, answer questions about your claim, and give you the names of participating physicians in your community. When writing to your carrier, be sure to include the word *Medicare* in the address.

If you are receiving railroad retirement benefits, your Medicare Part-B claims are handled by regional offices of the Travelers Insurance Company, regardless of your location. For the address and toll-free number of the office nearest you, call the Railroad Retirement Board, listed in your telephone directory under U.S. Government.

Alabama

Medicare
Blue Cross–Blue Shield
P.O. Box C-140
Birmingham, AL 35283
800-292-8855

Alaska

Medicare
Aetna Life and Casualty
200 S.W. Market Street
P.O. Box 1998
Portland, OR 97207
800-547-6333

Arizona

Medicare
Aetna Life and Casualty
P.O. Box 37200
Phoenix, AZ 85069
800-352-0411

Arkansas

Medicare
Arkansas Blue Cross and Blue
  Shield
P.O. Box 1418
Little Rock, AR 72203
800-482-5525

California

Counties of Los Angeles,
Orange, San Diego, Ventura,
Imperial, San Luis Obispo, and
Santa Barbara
  Medicare
  Transamerica Occidental Life
    Insurance Co.
  Box 50061
  Upland, CA 91785
  800-252-9020
Rest of the state:
  Medicare Claims Department
  Blue Shield of California
  Chico, CA 95976
  (from northern California)
    800-952-8627
  (from southern California)
    800-824-0900

Colorado

Medicare
Blue Shield of Colorado
700 Broadway
Denver, CO 80273
800-332-6681

Connecticut

Medicare
The Travelers Insurance
  Comapny
P.O. Box 5005
Wallingford, CN 64953
800-982-6783

Delaware

Medicare
Pennsylvania Blue Shield
P.O. Box 65
Camp Hill, PA 17011
800-851-3535

District of Columbia

Medicare
Pennsylvania Blue Shield
P.O. Box 100
Camp Hill, PA 17011
800-233-1124

Florida

Medicare
Blue Shield of Florida
P.O. Box 2525
Jacksonville, FL 32231
800-333-7586

Georgia

Medicare
Aetna Life and Casualty
P.O. Box 3018
Savannah, GA 31402
800-727-0827

Hawaii

Medicare
Aetna Life and Casualty
P.O. Box 3947
Honolulu, HI 96812
800-272-5242

Idaho

Medicare
EQUICOR, Inc.
P.O. Box 8048
Boise, ID 83707
800-632-6574

Illinois

Medicare Claims
Blue Cross and Blue Shield of
    Illinois
P.O. Box 4422
Marion, IL 62959
800-642-6930

Indiana

Medicare Part B
Associated Insurance
    Companies, Inc.
P.O. Box 7073
Indianapolis, IN 46207
800-622-4792

Iowa

Medicare
Blue Shield of Iowa
636 Grand
Des Moines, IA 50309
800-532-1285

Kansas

Counties of Johnson and
    Wyandotte:
Medicare
Blue Shield of Kansas City
P.O. Box 169
Kansas City, MO 64141
800-892-5900
Rest of the state:
Medicare
Blue Shield of Kansas
P.O. Box 239
Topeka, KS 66601
800-432-3531

Kentucky

Medicare Part B
Blue Cross and Blue Shield of
    Kentucky
100 East Vine Street
Lexington, KY 40507
800-432-9255

Louisiana

Medicare Administration
Blue Cross and Blue Shield of
    Louisiana
P.O. Box 95204
Baton Rouge, LA 70895
800-462-9666

Maine

Medicare
Blue Shield of Massachusetts/
    Tri-State
P.O. Box 1010
Biddeford, ME 04005
800-492-0919

Maryland

Counties of Montgomery and
Prince Georges:
  Medicare
  Pennsylvania Blue Shield
  P.O. Box 100
  Camp Hill, PA 17011
  800-233-1124
Rest of the state:
  Medicare
  Maryland Blue Shield
  700 E. Joppa Road
  Towson, MD 21204
  800-492-4795

Massachusetts

Medicare
Blue Shield of Massachusetts
55 Accord Park Drive
Rockland, MA 02371
800-882-1228

Michigan

Medicare Part B
Michigan Blue Cross and Blue
  Shield
P.O. Box 2201
Detroit, MI 48231
  (from area code 213)
    800-482-4045
  (from area code 517)
    800-322-0607
  (from area code 616)
    800-442-8020
  (from area code 906)
    800-562-7802
  (from Detroit)
    313-225-8200

Minnesota

Counties of Anoka, Dakota,
Filmore, Goodhue, Hennepin,
Houston, Olmstead, Ramsey,
Wabasha, Washington, and
Winona:
  Medicare
  The Travelers Insurance
    Company
  8120 Penn Avenue
  South Bloomington, MN
    55431
  800-352-2762
Rest of the state:
  Medicare
  Blue Shield of Minnesota
  P.O. Box 64357
  St. Paul, MN 55164
  800-392-0343

Mississippi

Medicare
The Travelers Insurance
  Company
P.O. Box 22545
Jackson, MS 39225
800-682-5417

Missouri

Counties of Andrew, Atchison,
Bates, Benton, Buchanan,
Caldwell, Carroll, Cass, Clay,
Clinton, Daviess, DeKalb,
Gentry, Grundy, Harrison,
Henry, Holt, Jackson, Johnson,
Lafayette, Livingston, Mercer,
Nodaway, Pettis, Platte, Ray, St.
Clair, Saline, Vernon, and
Worth:
  Medicare
  Blue Shield of Kansas City

P.O. Box 169
Kansas City, MO 64141
800-892-5900
Rest of the state:
Medicare
General American Life
  Insurance Company
P.O. Box 505
St. Louis, MO 63166
800-393-3070

Montana

Medicare
Blue Shield of Montana
2501 Beltview
P.O. Box 4310
Helena, MT 59604
800-332-6146

Nebraska

Medicare Part B
Blue Cross and Blue Shield of
  Nebraska
P.O. Box 3106
Omaha, NE 68103
800-633-1113

Nevada

Medicare
Aetna Life and Casualty
P.O. Box 37230
Phoenix, AZ 85069
800-528-0311

New Hampshire

Medicare
Blue Shield of Massachusetts/
  Tri-State
P.O. Box 1010
Biddeford, ME 04005
800-447-1142

New Jersey

Medicare
Pennsylvania Blue Shield
P.O. Box 400010
Harrisburg, PA 17140
800-462-9306

New Mexico

Medicare
Aetna Life and Casualty
P.O. Box 25500
Oklahoma City, OK 73125
800-423-2925

New York

Counties of Bronx, Columbia,
Delaware, Dutchess, Greene,
Kings, Nassau, New York,
Orange, Putnam, Richmond,
Rockland, Suffolk, Sullivan,
Ulster, and Westchester:
  Medicare
  Empire Blue Cross and Blue
    Shield
  P.O. Box 100
  Yorktown Heights, NY 10598
  800-442-8430
County of Queens:
  Medicare
  Group Health, Inc.
  P.O. Box A966
  Times Square Station
  New York, NY 10036
  800-252-6550
Rest of the state:
  Blue Shield of Western
    New York
  P.O. Box 0600
  Binghamton, NY 13902
  800-252-6550

North Carolina

Medicare
EQUICOR, Inc.
P.O. Box 671
Nashville, TN 37202
800-672-3071

North Dakota

Medicare
Blue Shield of North Dakota
4510 13th Avenue, S.W.
Fargo, ND 58121
800-247-2267

Ohio

Medicare
Nationwide Mutual Insurance
    Company
P.O. Box 57
Columbus, OH 43216
800-282-0530

Oklahoma

Medicare
Aetna Life and Casualty
701 N.W. 63rd Street, Suite 300
Oklahoma City, OK 73116
800-522-9079

Oregon

Medicare
Aetna Life and Casualty
200 S.W. Market Street
P.O. Box 1997
Portland, OR 97207
503-222-6831

Pennsylvania

Medicare
Pennsylvania Blue Shield
Box 65
Camp Hill, PA 17011
800-382-1274

Rhode Island

Medicare
Blue Shield of Rhode Island
444 Westminster Mall
Providence, RI 02901
800-662-5170

South Carolina

Medicare Part B
Blue Cross and Blue Shield of
    South Carolina
Fontaine Road Business Center
300 Arbor Lake Drive, Suite
    1300
Columbia, SC 29223
800-922-2340

South Dakota

Medicare Part B
Blue Shield of North Dakota
4510 13th Avenue, S.W.
Fargo, ND 58121
800-437-4762

Tennessee

Medicare
EQUICOR, Inc.
P.O. Box 1465
Nashville, TN 37202
800-342-8900

Texas

Medicare
Blue Cross and Blue Shield of
  Texas
P.O. Box 660031
Dallas, TX 75266
800-442-2620

Utah

Medicare
Blue Shield of Utah
P.O. Box 30269
2455 Parley's Way
Salt Lake City, UT 84130
800-426-3477

Vermont

Medicare
Blue Shield of Massachusetts/
  Tri-State
P.O. Box 1010
Biddeford, ME 04005
800-447-1142

Virginia

Counties of Arlington and
  Fairfax:
Cities of Alexandria, Falls
  Church, and Fairfax:
Medicare
Pennsylvania Blue Shield
P.O. Box 100
Camp Hill, PA 17011
800-233-1124
Rest of the state:
Medicare
The Travelers Insurance Co.
P.O. Box 26463
Richmond, VA 23261
800-254-4130

Washington

Mail claims to your local Medical
Service Bureau. If you do not
know which bureau handles
your claim, mail it to:

Medicare
Washington Physicians' Service
4th and Battery Bldg., 6th Floor
2401 4th Avenue
Seattle, WA 98121
(from King County) 800-422-4087
(from Spokane)   800-572-5256
(from Kitsap)   800-552-7114
(from Pierce)   206-597-6530

West Virginia

Medicare
Nationwide Mutual Insurance
  Co.
P.O. Box 57
Columbus, OH 43216
800-848-0106

Wisconsin

Medicare
Wisconsin Physicians' Service
Box 1787
Madison, WI 53701
800-362-7221

Wyoming

Medicare
EQUICOR, Inc.
P.O. Box 628
Indian Hills Shopping Center
Cheyenne, WY 82003
800-442-2371

American Samoa

Medicare
Hawaii Medical Services
  Association
818 Keeaumoku Street
Honolulu, HI 96808
800-944-2247

Guam

Medicare
Aetna Life and Casualty
P.O. Box 3947
Honolulu, HI 96812
808-524-1240

Northern Mariana Islands

Medicare
Aetna Life and Casualty
P.O. Box 3947
Honolulu, HI 96812
808-524-1240

Puerto Rico

Medicare
Seguros de Servicio de Salud de
  Puerto Rico
Call Box 71391
San Juan, PR 00936
800-462-7385

Virgin Islands

Medicare
Seguros de Servicio de Salud de
  Puerto Rico
Call Box 71391
San Juan, PR 00936
800-462-2970

Appendix B:
Where to Go for Help

If you have a problem about health-care insurance, the agencies listed in this section may be able to help. Every state has an:

1. **Insurance commissioner,** whose job is to regulate insurance companies and agents. Insurance commissioners have the power to stop unfair and deceptive sales practices. Some also provide booklets and other materials that help consumers compare policies sold in their state.
2. **Attorney general,** who is responsible for enforcing anti-fraud and consumer protection laws. In most states, the attorney general can file suit to stop illegal practices by insurance companies, agents, and health-care providers.
3. **Agency on aging,** which oversees the activities of local agencies that provide health, housing, nutrition, legal, and other services for older Americans. Your state agency on aging can give you the name and address of the agency serving your area.

Some communities have **health insurance counseling programs** that help seniors with problems with Medicare, Medicaid, and supplemental health-care insurance. There are also **senior legal services programs** that assist when legal advice or representation is needed. Both programs can help you deal with such problems as abusive sales practices, aggressive medical bill collectors, and the process of appealing decisions about Medicare claims. Your state insurance commissioner or state agency on aging should know whether any such programs serve your area.

Alabama

Insurance Commissioner
135 South Union Street, #160
Montgomery, AL 36130
205-269-3550

Attorney General of Alabama
State Capitol
11 South Union Street
Montgomery, AL 36130
205-261-7300

State Agency on Aging
136 Catoma Street
Montgomery, AL 36130
205-261-5743

Alaska

Director of Insurance
333 Willoughby Avenue, 9th
  Floor
Juneau, AK 99811
907-465-2515

Attorney General of Alaska
P.O. Box K, State Capitol
Juneau, AK 99811
907-465-3600

Older Alaskans Commission
P.O. Box C, MS 0209
Juneau, AK 99811
907-465-3250

Arizona

Insurance Commissioner
3030 North 3rd Street, Suite
  1100
Phoenix, AZ 85012
602-255-5400

Attorney General of Arizona
1275 West Washington Street
Phoenix, AZ 85007
602-255-4266

Aging and Adult Administration
Department of Economic
  Security
1400 West Washington Street
Phoenix, AZ 85007
602-255-4446

Arkansas

Insurance Commissioner
400 University Tower Bldg.
12th and University Streets
Little Rock, AR 72204
501-371-1325

Attorney General of Arkansas
200 Tower Building
4th and Center Streets
Little Rock, AR 72201
501-682-2007

State Agency on Aging
Donaghey Bldg., Suite 1428
Main and 7th Streets
Little Rock, AR 72201
501-682-2441

California

Insurance Commissioner
Northern California Office
100 Van Ness Avenue
San Francisco, CA 94102
415-557-9624

Insurance Commissioner
Southern California Office
3540 Wilshire Blvd.
Los Angeles, CA 90010
213-736-2572

Attorney General of California
1515 K Street, Suite 638
Sacramento, CA 95814
916-445-9555

California Department on Aging
1600 K Street
Sacramento, CA 95814
916-322-3887

Health Insurance Counseling
and Advocacy Program
1600 K Street
Sacramento, CA 95814
916-323-7315

Colorado

Insurance Commissioner
303 West Colfax Avenue, 5th
Floor
Denver, CO 80204
303-620-4300

Attorney General of Colorado
1525 Sherman Street, 2nd Floor
Denver, CO 80203
303-866-5005

Aging and Adult Services
Department of Social Services
1575 Sherman Street, 10th Floor
Denver, CO 80203
303-866-5905

Connecticut

Insurance Commissioner
165 Capitol Avenue
State Office Bldg., Room 425
Hartford, CT 06106
203-297-3801

Attorney General of Connecticut
Capitol Annex
30 Trinity Street
Hartford, CT 06106
203-566-2026

State Agency on Aging
175 Main Street
Hartford, CT 06106
203-566-3238

Delaware

Insurance Commissioner
841 Silver Lake Blvd.
Dover, DE 19901
302-736-4251

Attorney General of Delaware
820 North French Street
8th Floor
Wilmington, DE 19801
302-571-3838

Delaware Division on Aging
Department of Health and
Social Services
1901 North Dupont Highway
New Castle, DE 19720
302-421-6791

District of Columbia

Insurance Commissioner
613 G Street, N.W.
6th Floor
Washington, DC 20001
202-727-7424

Corporation Counsel of the
  District of Columbia
1350 Pennsylvania Avenue,
  N.W.
Suite 329
Washington, DC 20004
202-727-6248

Office on Aging
Executive Office of the Mayor
1424 K Street, N.W.
2nd Floor
Washington, DC 20005
202-724-5622

Florida

Insurance Commissioner
State Capitol
Plaza Level Eleven
Tallahassee, FL 32399
904-488-3440

Attorney General of Florida
State Capitol
Tallahassee, FL 32399
904-487-1963

State Agency on Aging
Department of Health and
  Rehabilitative Services
Building 2, Room 323
1323 Winewood Blvd.
Tallahassee, FL 32399
904-488-8922

Georgia

Insurance Commissioner
2 Martin Luther King Drive
Floyd Memorial Bldg.
704 West Tower
Atlanta, GA 30334
404-656-2056

Attorney General of Georgia
132 State Judicial Bldg.
Atlanta, GA 30334
404-656-4585

Office on Aging
Department of Human
  Resources
6th Floor
878 Peachtree Street, N.E.
Atlanta, GA 30309
404-894-5333

Hawaii

Insurance Commissioner
1010 Richards Street
Honolulu, HI 96813
808-548-5450

Attorney General of Hawaii
State Capitol, Room 405
Honolulu, HI 96813
808-548-4740

Hawaii Executive Office on
  Aging
335 Merchant Street, Room 241
Honolulu, HI 96813
808-548-2593

Idaho

Director of Insurance
500 South 10th Street
Boise, ID 83720
208-334-2250

Attorney General of Idaho
State House
Boise, ID 83720
208-334-2400

Office on Aging
State House, Room 114
Boise, ID 83720
208-334-3833

Senior Health Insurance
Benefits Advisors
Idaho Department of Insurance
500 South 10th Street
Boise, ID 83720
208-334-2250

Illinois

Insurance Commissioner
State of Illinois Center
100 West Randolph Street
Suite 15-100
Chicago, IL 60601
312-917-2420

Attorney General of Illinois
100 West Randolph Street
12th Floor
Chicago, IL 60601
312-917-3000

Department on Aging
421 East Capitol Avenue
Springfield, IL 62701
217-785-2870

Senior Health Insurance
Program
Illinois Department of Insurance
320 West Washington Street
Springfield, IL 62767
217-782-0004

Indiana

Insurance Commissioner
311 West Washington Street
Suite 300
Indianapolis, IN 46204
317-232-2386

Attorney General of Indiana
219 State House
Indianapolis, IN 46204
317-232-6201

Indiana Department of Human
Services
251 North Illinois
P.O. Box 7083
Indianapolis, IN 46207
317-232-1139

Iowa

Insurance Commissioner
Lucas State Office Bldg.
6th Floor
Des Moines, IA 50319
515-281-5705

Attorney General of Iowa
Hoover Bldg.
2nd Floor
Des Moines, IA 50319
515-281-5164

Department of Elder Affairs
Jewett Bldg., Suite 236
914 Grand Avenue
Des Moines, IA 50319
515-281-5187

Protection and Advocacy
Through Community
Training

Iowa Insurance Division
Lucas State Office Building
6th Floor
Des Moines, IA 50319
515-242-5190

Kansas

Insurance Commissioner
420 S.W. 9th Street
Topeka, KS 66612
913-296-7801

Attorney General of Kansas
Judicial Center, 2nd Floor
Topeka, KS 66612
913-296-2215

Department on Aging
610 West Tenth Street
Topeka, KS 66612
913-296-4986

Kentucky

Insurance Commissioner
229 West Main Street
Frankfort, KY 40602
502-564-3630

Attorney General of Kentucky
State Capitol, Room 116
Frankfort, KY 40601
502-564-7600

Division for Aging Services
Department for Social Services
275 East Main Street
Frankfort, KY 40621
502-564-6930

Louisiana

Insurance Commissioner
950 North 5th Street
Baton Rouge, LA 70801
504-342-5328

Attorney General of Louisiana
2-3-4 Loyola Bldg.
New Orleans, LA 70112
504-568-5575

Governor's Office of Elderly
   Affairs
P.O. Box 80374
Baton Rouge, LA 70898
504-925-1700

Maine

Superintendent of Insurance
State Office Bldg.
State House
Station 34
Augusta, ME 04333
207-582-8707

Attorney General of Maine
State House
Augusta, ME 04330
207-289-3661

Bureau of Maine's Elderly
Department of Human Services
State House
Station 11
Augusta, ME 04333
207-289-2561

Maryland

Insurance Commissioner
501 St. Paul Place
Stanbalt Bldg., 7th Floor South
Baltimore, MD 21202
301-333-2520

Attorney General of Maryland
Munsey Bldg.
Calvert and Fayette Streets
Baltimore, MD 21202
301-576-6300

Maryland Office on Aging
301 West Preston Street
Baltimore, MD 21201
301-225-1102

Senior Health Insurance
   Counseling Program
301 West Preston Street
Baltimore, MD 21201
301-225-1270

Massachusetts

Insurance Commissioner
280 Friend Street
Boston, MA 02114
617-727-7189

Attorney General of
   Massachusetts
One Ashburton Place,
   20th Floor
Boston, MA 02108
617-727-2200

Massachusetts Executive Office
   of Elder Affairs
38 Chauncey Street
Boston, MA 02111
617-727-7750

Serving Health Information
   Needs of Elders
38 Chauncey Street
Boston, MA 02111
617-727-7750

Michigan

Insurance Commissioner
611 West Ottawa Street
2nd Floor North
Lansing, MI 48933
517-373-9273

Attorney General of Michigan
Law Bldg.
525 West Ottawa Street
Lansing, MI 48913
517-373-1110

Office of Services to the Aging
P.O. Box 30026
Lansing, MI 48909
517-373-8230

Minnesota

Insurance Commissioner
500 Metro Square Bldg.
5th Floor
St. Paul, MN 55101
612-296-6848

Attorney General of Minnesota
102 State Capitol
St. Paul, MN 55155
612-296-6196

Minnesota Board of Aging
Metro Square Bldg., Suite 204
7th and Robert Streets
St. Paul, MN 55101
612-296-2770

Mississippi

Insurance Commissioner
1804 Walter Sillers Bldg.
Jackson, MS 39205
601-359-3569

Attorney General of Mississippi
P.O. Box 220
Jackson, MS 39205
601-359-3680

Mississippi Council on Aging
301 West Pearl Street
Jackson, MS 39203
601-949-2070

Missouri

Director of Insurance
301 West High Street 6 North
Jefferson City, MO 65102
314-751-2451

Attorney General of Missouri
Supreme Court Bldg.
101 High Street
Jefferson City, MO 65102
314-751-3321

Division on Aging
Department of Social Services
2701 West Main Street
P.O. Box 1337
Jefferson City, MO 65102
314-751-3082

Montana

Insurance Commissioner
Mitchell Bldg., Room 270
126 North Sanders
Helena, MT 59601
406-444-2040

Attorney General of Montana
Justice Bldg.
215 North Sanders
Helena, MT 59620
406-444-2026

Department of Family Services
P.O. Box 8005
Helena, MT 59604
406-444-5900

Nebraska

Director of Insurance
Terminal Bldg., Suite 400
941 "O" Street
Lincoln, NE 68508
402-471-2201

Attorney General of Nebraska
2115 State Capitol
Lincoln, NE 68509
402-471-2682

Department on Aging
301 Centennial Mall South
Lincoln, NE 68509
402-471-2306

Nevada

Insurance Commissioner
Wye Bldg.
201 South Fall Street
Carson City, NV 89710
702-885-4270

Attorney General of Nevada
Heroes Memorial Bldg.
Capitol Complex
Carson City, NV 89710
702-687-4170

Nevada Division for Aging
  Services
Department of Human
  Resources
505 East King Street, Room 101
Carson City, NV 89710
702-885-4210

New Hampshire

Insurance Commissioner
169 Manchester Street
Concord, NH 03301
603-271-2261

Attorney General of
New Hampshire
208 State House Annex
Concord, NH 03301
603-271-3658

Division of Elderly and Adult
Services
6 Hazen Drive
Concord, NH 03301
603-271-4390

New Jersey

Insurance Commissioner
20 West State Street CN 325
Trenton, NJ 08625
609-292-5363

Attorney General of New Jersey
Richard J. Hughes Justice
Complex CN 080
Trenton, NJ 08625
609-292-4925

New Jersey Division on Aging
South Broad and Front Streets
CN 807
Trenton, NJ 08625
609-292-0920

Senior Health Insurance
Program
Division on Aging
CN 807
Trenton, NJ 08625
609-292-4303

New Mexico

Superintendent of Insurance
PERA Bldg., 4th Floor
500 Old Santa Fe Trail
Santa Fe, NM 87501
505-827-4500

Attorney General of
New Mexico
Bataan Memorial Bldg.
Galisteo Street
Santa Fe, NM 87503
505-827-6000

Agency on Aging
La Villa Rivera Bldg., 4th Floor
223 East Palace Avenue
Santa Fe, NM 87501
505-827-7640

Health Insurance Benefits
Assistance Program
224 East Palace Avenue
4th Floor
Santa Fe, NM 87501
505-827-7640

New York

Superintendent of Insurance
160 West Broadway
New York, NY 10013
212-602-0249

Attorney General of New York
120 West Broadway, 25th Floor
New York, NY 10271
212-341-2519

New York State Office for the
Aging
Agency Bldg. #2
Empire State Plaza
Albany, NY 12223
518-474-5731

North Carolina

Insurance Commissioner
Dobbs Bldg.
430 Salisbury Street
Raleigh, NC 27611
919-733-7439

Attorney General of North
  Carolina
Department of Justice
2 East Morgan Street
Raleigh, NC 27602
919-733-3377

Division on Aging
Department of Human
  Resources
Kirby Bldg.
1985 Umstead Drive
Raleigh, NC 27603
919-733-3983

Senior Health Insurance
  Information Program
P.O. Box 26387
Raleigh, NC 27611
919-733-0433

North Dakota

Insurance Commissioner
Capitol Bldg., 5th Floor
Bismarck, ND 58505
701-224-2440

Attorney General of
  North Dakota
Department of Justice
2115 State Capitol
Bismarck, ND 58505
701-224-2210

Aging Services Division
Department of Human Services
State Capitol Bldg.
Bismarck, ND 58505
701-224-2577

Ohio

Director of Insurance
2100 Stella Court
Columbus, OH 43266
614-644-2658

Attorney General of Ohio
State Office Tower
30 East Broad Street
Columbus, OH 43266
614-466-3376

Ohio Department of Aging
50 West Broad Street, 9th Floor
Columbus, OH 43266
614-466-5500

Health Insurance Information
  Program for Older Adults
Office of the Attorney General
State Office Tower
30 East Broad Street
Columbus, OH 43215
614-466-8600

Oklahoma

Insurance Commissioner
1901 North Walnut
Oklahoma City, OK 73105
405-521-2828

Attorney General of Oklahoma
112 State Capitol
Oklahoma City, OK 73105
405-521-3921

Division of Aging Services
Department of Human Services
P.O. Box 25352
Oklahoma City, OK 73125
405-521-2327

Oregon

Insurance Commissioner
21 Labor and Industries Bldg.
Salem, OR 97310
503-378-4271

Attorney General of Oregon
100 Justice Bldg.
Salem, OR 97310
503-378-6002

Senior Services Division
Department of Human
　Resources
313 Public Services Bldg.
Salem, OR 97310
503-378-4728

Pennsylvania

Insurance Commissioner
Strawberry Square, 13th Floor
Harrisburg, PA 17120
717-787-5173

Attorney General of
　Pennsylvania
Strawberry Square, 16th Floor
Harrisburg, PA 17120
717-787-3391

Pennsylvania Department of
　Aging
Barto Bldg.
231 State Street
Harrisburg, PA 17101
717-783-1550

Rhode Island

Insurance Commissioner
233 Richmond Street, Suite 237
Providence, RI 02903
401-277-2246

Attorney General of
　Rhode Island
72 Pine Street
Providence, RI 02903
401-274-4400

Department of Elderly Affairs
79 Washington Street
Providence, RI 02903
401-277-2858

South Carolina

Insurance Commissioner
1612 Marion Street
Columbia, SC 29201
803-737-6117

Attorney General of South
　Carolina
Rembert Dennis Office Bldg.
1000 Assembly Street
Columbia, SC 29211
803-734-3970

South Carolina Commission on
　Aging
400 Arbor Lake Drive,
　Suite B-500
Columbia, SC 29223
803-735-0210

South Dakota

Director of Insurance
Insurance Bldg.
910 East Sioux Avenue
Pierre, SD 57501
605-773-3563

Attorney General of
  South Dakota
State Capitol Bldg.
Pierre, SD 57501
605-773-3215

Adult Services and Aging
700 Governors Drive
Pierre, SD 57501
605-773-3656

Tennessee

Insurance Commissioner
Volunteer Plaza
500 James Robertson Parkway
Nashville, TN 37219
615-741-2241

Attorney General of Tennessee
450 James Robertson Parkway
Nashville, TN 37219
615-741-3491

Tennessee Commission on
  Aging
706 Church Street, Suite 201
Nashville, TN 37219
615-741-2056

Texas

State Board of Insurance
1110 San Jacinto Blvd.
Austin, TX 78701
512-463-6330

Attorney General of Texas
P.O. Box 12548
Capitol Station
Austin, TX 78711
512-463-2100

Texas Department on Aging
P.O. Box 12786
Capitol Station
Austin, TX 78711
512-444-2727

Utah

Insurance Commissioner
Heber M. Wells Bldg.
160 East Third Street
Salt Lake City, UT 84145
801-530-6400

Attorney General of Utah
236 State Capitol
Salt Lake City, UT 84114
801-538-1015

Utah Division of Aging and
  Adult Services
P.O. Box 45500
Salt Lake City, UT 84145
801-538-3910

Vermont

Insurance Commissioner
State Office Bldg.
Montpelier, VT 05602
802-828-3301

Attorney General of Vermont
Pavillion Office Bldg.
Montpelier, VT 05602
802-828-3171

Vermont Office on Aging
Waterbury Complex
103 South Main Street
Waterbury, VT 05676
802-241-2400

Virginia

Insurance Commissioner
700 Jefferson Bldg.
1220 Bank Street
Richmond, VA 23219
804-774-2991

Attorney General of Virginia
101 North 8th Street, 5th Floor
Richmond, VA 23219
804-786-2071

Virginia Department for the
    Aging
101 North 14th Street,
    18th Floor
Richmond, VA 23219
804-225-2271

Washington

Insurance Commissioner
Insurance Bldg. AQ21
Olympia, WA 98504
206-753-7301

Attorney General of Washington
Highways-Licenses Bldg. PB71
Olympia, WA 98504
206-753-6200

Aging and Adult Services
    Administration
Mail Stop OB44A
Olympia, WA 98504
206-586-3768

Senior Health Insurance
    Benefits Advisors
Insurance Building
Olympia, WA 98504
206-753-2408

West Virginia

Insurance Commissioner
2019 Washington Street East
Charleston, WV 25305
304-348-3394

Attorney General of West
    Virginia
State Capitol
Charleston, WV 25305
304-348-2021

West Virginia Commission on
    Aging
State Capitol Complex
Holly Grove
Charleston, WV 25305
304-348-3317

Wisconsin

Insurance Commissioner
123 West Washington Avenue
Madison, WI 53702
608-266-0102

Attorney General of Wisconsin
State Capitol, 114 East
Madison, WI 53707
608-266-1221

Bureau on Aging
P.O. Box 7851
Madison, WI 53707
608-266-2536

Wyoming

Insurance Commissioner
Herschler Bldg.
122 West 25th Street
Cheyenne, WY 82002
307-777-7401

Attorney General of Wyoming
123 State Capitol
Cheyenne, WY 82002
307-777-7841

Commission on Aging
Hathaway Bldg. 1st Floor
Cheyenne, WY 82002
307-777-7986

American Samoa

Insurance Commissioner
Office of the Governor
Pago Pago, American Samoa
96797
684-633-4116

Attorney General of American
Samoa
P.O. Box 7
Pago Pago, American Samoa
96799
684-633-4163

Territorial Administration on
Aging
Government of American Samoa
Pago Pago, American Samoa
96799
684-633-1251

Guam

Insurance Commissioner
855 West Marine Drive
Agana, Guam 96910
671-477-1040

Attorney General of Guam
Department of Law
238 F. C. Flores Street, #701
Agana, Guam 96910
671-472-6841

Division of Senior Citizens
P.O. Box 2816
Agana, Guam 96910
671-734-2942

Northern Mariana Islands

Attorney General of the
Northern Mariana Islands
Saipan, CM 96950
670-234-6207

Department of Community and
Cultural Affairs
Civic Center
Saipan, CM 96950
670-234-6011

Puerto Rico

Insurance Commissioner
Fernandez Juncos Station
Santurce, PR 00910
809-722-8686

Attorney General of Puerto Rico
Department of Justice
P.O. Box 192
San Juan, PR 00902
809-721-2900

Puerto Rico Gericulture
Commission
Department of Social Services
Box 11398
Santurce, PR 00910
809-724-1059

Virgin Islands

Insurance Commissioner
Kongens Gade #18
St. Thomas, VI 00802
809-774-2991

Attorney General of the Virgin
  Islands
Department of Justice
Norre Gade #46
U.S. Post Office Bldg.,
  2nd Floor
St. Thomas, VI 00801
809-774-5666

Senior Citizens Affairs
Department of Human Services
6F Haversight Mall
Charlotte Amalie
St. Thomas, VI 00801
809-774-5884

Appendix C:
Worksheets, Sample Letters, and Forms

Medicare Supplement Insurance Worksheets

Hospital Services

Do you need a private nurse and/or private room even when those services are not medically necessary?

Yes _____ No _____

- If yes, investigate policies with private nursing or private room coverage.
- If no, consider policies without this coverage.

Do you have any special conditions that will require more than 100 days of care in a skilled nursing facility?

Yes _____ No _____

- If yes, investigate policies with extended skilled-nursing coverage. Many supplement policies cover the $74 per day co-payment for the 21st through 100th day you are in a skilled nursing facility. In addition, some will pay for care after Medicare coverage ends on the 100th day.
- If no, consider policies without extended skilled nursing coverage.

Doctors' Services

Have all of your doctors agreed to accept Medicare assignment?

Yes _____   No _____

Can you find doctors in your area who will agree to accept Medicare assignment?

Yes _____   No _____

- Consult the table in Appendix D to find out what percent of the doctors in your state accept Medicare assignment for all services they provide to Medicare patients. Also, check with your Medicare insurance carrier for the names and addresses of "Participating Physicians" in your area.

Are you willing to switch to doctors who have agreed to accept assignment?

Yes _____   No _____

- If the answers to these questions are no, investigate policies that will pay for all or some of any charges in excess of Medicare-approved amounts.
- If your answers to these questions are yes, consider policies without this coverage.

Other Services

Do you need routine eye, hearing, foot, or dental care more than a few times a year?

Yes _____   No _____

Do you spend more than $75 a year on prescription drugs?

Yes _____   No _____

Do you plan to travel outside the United States?

Yes _____   No _____

- If the answer to any of these questions is yes, investigate policies that provide the relevant coverage.

- If your answers are no, these features are not important to you. Consider policies without these extras.

Your Health

Are you in good health and under age 70?

Yes _____   No _____

- If yes, consider companies that charge lower premiums for "preferred risks," or companies that accept only healthy applicants.
- If no, consider companies that charge everyone the same rate and do not rigorously screen out applicants because of poor health.

Do you have a medical condition that needs ongoing treatment, or may need treatment at any time?

Yes _____   No _____

- If yes, look for a policy that will cover pre-existing conditions immediately, or purchase a rider that will provide you with that coverage.
- If no, consider policies that have a waiting period before covering pre-existing conditions.

Protection Against Cancellation

Are you willing to save money if it means buying a policy that could be canceled by the company?

Yes _____   No _____

- If yes, consider policies without any protection against cancellation. Keep in mind that companies often exercise their right to cancel policies.
- If no, consider guaranteed renewable or conditionally renewable policies.

Health Maintenance Organizations

Are there any Health Maintenance Organizations (HMOs) in your area that provide care to Medicare beneficiaries? (To find out, contact a Social Security office.)

Yes _____ No _____

- If yes, investigate them further. An HMO may be a cost-effective alternative to buying a Medicare supplement policy.
- If no, review this worksheet before shopping for a policy.

FORM APPROVED
OMB NO. 0938-0008

PATIENT'S REQUEST FOR MEDICAL PAYMENT

IMPORTANT—SEE OTHER SIDE FOR INSTRUCTIONS

MEDICAL INSURANCE BENEFITS SOCIAL SECURITY ACT

PLEASE TYPE OR PRINT INFORMATION

NOTICE: Anyone who misrepresents or falsifies essential information requested by this form may upon conviction be subject to fine and imprisonment under Federal Law. No Part B Medicare benefits may be paid unless this form is received as required by existing law and regulations (20 CFR 422.510).

SEND COMPLETED FORM TO:

1. Name of Beneficiary from Health Insurance Card
   (Last)   (First)   (Middle)

2. Claim Number from Health Insurance Card

   Patient's Sex
   ☐ Male
   ☐ Female

3. Patient's Mailing Address (City, State, Zip Code)
   Check here if this is a new address ☐

   (Street or P.O. Box — Include Apartment Number)

   (City)   (State)   (Zip)

   3b. Telephone Number
   (Include Area Code)
   (———) ——— ———

4. Describe the Illness or Injury for which Patient Received Treatment

   4b. Was condition related to:
   A. Patient's employment
   ☐ Yes   ☐ No

   B. Accident
   ☐ Auto   ☐ Other

4c Was patient being treated with chronic dialysis or kidney transplant?
☐ Yes ☐ No

5

a. Are you employed and covered under an employee health plan?
☐ Yes ☐ No

b. Is your spouse employed and are you covered under your spouse's employee health plan?
☐ Yes ☐ No

c. If you have any medical coverage other than Medicare, such as private insurance, employment related insurance, State Agency (Medicaid), or the VA, complete:
Name and Address of other insurance, State Agency (Medicaid), or VA office

Policyholders Name:

Policy or Medical Assistance No.

NOTE: If you DO NOT want payment information on this claim released, put an (X) here ⟶ ☐

I AUTHORIZE ANY HOLDER OF MEDICAL OR OTHER INFORMATION ABOUT ME TO RELEASE TO THE SOCIAL SECURITY ADMINISTRATION AND HEALTH CARE FINANCING ADMINISTRATION OR ITS INTERMEDIARIES OR CARRIERS ANY INFORMATION NEEDED FOR THIS OR A RELATED MEDICARE CLAIM. I PERMIT A COPY OF THIS AUTHORIZATION TO BE USED IN PLACE OF THE ORIGINAL, AND REQUEST PAYMENT OF MEDICAL INSURANCE BENEFITS TO ME.

6

Signature of Patient (If patient is unable to sign, see Block 6 on reverse)

6b Date signed

IMPORTANT
ATTACH ITEMIZED BILLS FROM YOUR DOCTOR(S) OR SUPPLIER(S) TO THE BACK OF THIS FORM
DEPARTMENT OF HEALTH AND HUMAN SERVICES—HEALTH CARE FINANCING ADMINISTRATION

Form HCFA-1490S (SC) (2-87)

Sample Letter Canceling a Medicare Supplement Policy

In most states, you have 30 days from the time you receive a policy to review it and return it to the company for a full refund. If you decide you don't want the policy, write a letter canceling the policy and send it by registered mail so that you will have proof that it was delivered within the 30-day period. Use the following sample letter as a starting point and adapt it, if necessary, to your particular situation.

[Date]

Dear [insert name of insurance company]:

On [insert date you received policy], I received [name of policy and policy number] from your company. I have carefully reviewed the policy and have decided that I do not want the insurance.

Therefore, I am exercising my right to cancel the policy and request that you refund the $[insert amount] that I paid on [insert date]. Enclosed is the policy that I received. I will appreciate a prompt refund of my premium. Thank you for your assistance.

Sincerely,

[Your Name]

encl. Medicare Supplement Policy

Sample Letter to the State Insurance Commissioner

If an insurance company refuses to refund all of your premium, send the following letter to your state insurance commissioner. If the commissioner is slow in responding to your letter, send a similar letter to the state attorney general. (See Appendix B for addresses.)

[Date]

Dear Commissioner:

The purpose of this letter is to file a formal complaint against [insert name of insurance company]. On [insert date you received policy], I received [policy name, policy number]. I canceled the policy on [date you returned the policy to the company] within the 30-day cancellation period provided under state law.

The company has failed to respond to my letter [or describe its response—for example, "On June 11, 1990, I received a letter from the company stating that it was refunding only $25 of the $250 I paid for the policy"].

Please look into this matter to ensure that the company complies with its legal obligation to refund my entire premium. I have enclosed a copy of my cancellation letter to the company [if necessary, add, "and the letter I received from the company"].

If you need more information, please contact me. Please let me know the results of your investigation. Thank you for your assistance.

Sincerely,

[Your Name]

encl. Copy of cancellation letter
[If necessary, include copy of company's reply]

Sample Letter Appealing a Claims Decision

To appeal a claims decision, you can simply write a letter to the Medicare insurance carrier requesting an appeal. Use the following letter to make the initial request and obtain documents on which the claims decision was based. You can adapt the letter for subsequent steps in the appeal process.

[Date]

Dear [insert name of carrier]:

I am formally appealing the denial of my claim dated [insert claim date]. I do not agree with the decision reached on my claim because [give reason—for example, "the home health services I received are covered by Medicare"].

So that I may adequately present evidence supporting my appeal, I would appreciate it if you would provide me with copies of the rules that were applied in denying my claim, and all of the documents contained in my claim file.

For your reference, my Medicare identification number is [insert number], and I enclose a copy of the EOMB denying my claim. Thank you for your assistance.

Sincerely,

[Your Name]

encl.

Sample Letter Requesting a Refund from a Doctor

If Medicare denies a claim because it finds that the services provided were not medically necessary, the doctor or other provider may be required to refund the amount you paid for those services. Use the following letter to request a refund.

[Date]

Dear Dr. [insert doctor's name]:

The purpose of this letter is to request that you refund the $[insert amount] I paid for [state the operation, procedure, or service you received—for example, "the laetrile treatments you performed in June"].

Recently, I was notified by Medicare that they consider that the treatments were not medically necessary. As you know, neither you nor your staff informed me in advance that Medicare was unlikely to pay for this procedure, nor did I ever agree to pay under those circumstances. Had you told me, I would not have gone ahead with the treatments.

I have been notified that federal law requires that you make a prompt refund of the money I paid you. I shall expect to receive a refund of the full amount from you within 30 days; otherwise, I will be forced to file a formal complaint with both Medicare and law enforcement agencies. Thank you for your cooperation.

Sincerely,

[Your Name]

Sample Letter to a Law Enforcement Agency

If the doctor or other health-care provider fails to refund your money, use the following letter to request help from your Medicare carrier and your state attorney general. (The addresses are listed in Appendix A and Appendix B.)

[Date]

Dear [insert name]:

The purpose of this letter is to file a formal complaint against Dr. [insert full name and address]. [Describe the services you received from the doctor and how much you paid. For example, "In June of this year, the doctor prescribed several treatments involving the drug laetrile. For those treatments, I paid him a total of $2,550."]

Neither the doctor nor his staff informed me in advance that Medicare was unlikely to pay for this procedure. Nor did I ever agree to pay for the treatments under those circumstances. Had the doctor told me that Medicare would consider these treatments unreasonable and unnecessary, I would have refused to go ahead with the treatments.

On [insert date], I received a notice from Medicare (copy enclosed) denying my claim, stating that those treatments are not considered to be reasonable and necessary. On [insert date], I wrote to the doctor and informed him of Medicare's determination and requested a prompt refund of the amount I paid him. I enclose a copy of that letter.

To date, the doctor has not refunded my money. [Describe the doctor's response. For example, "Several weeks after I wrote him, his office manager telephoned me and said that since I received the treatments, the doctor will not be refunding my money."].

I understand that the doctor's actions are a violation of federal law. Please look into this matter. If you need more information, please contact me. I look forward to hearing the results of your investigation.

Sincerely,

[Your Name]

encl. [Copies of EOMB and your letter to the doctor.]

In addition to sending the preceding letter, also report the problem to the inspector general of the U.S. Department of Health and Human Services. That office is responsible for conducting investigations into fraud and abuse by health-care providers. Investigations can lead to both civil and criminal penalties and exclusion from the Medicare program. The inspector general maintains a hotline to receive evidence of fraud and abuse. The toll-free number is 800-368-5779 (from Maryland: 800-638-3986).

Sample Explanation of Medical Benefits (EOMB)

YOUR EXPLANATION OF MEDICARE BENEFITS

READ THIS NOTICE CAREFULLY AND
KEEP IT FOR YOUR RECORDS. THIS IS NOT A BILL.

HEALTH CARE FINANCING
ADMINISTRATION

APRIL 27, 1990

Need help? Contact:

JOHN DOE
STREET ADDRESS
CITY, STATE, ZIP COPE

Medicare Claims Dept.
Carrier's Name
Carrier's Address
Telephone: 800-123-4567

STATEMENT NUMBER 028607242-1 CHECK NUMBER 0814755259

Assignment was not taken on your claim for $145.00. (See item 4 on the back.)

Claim Control Number ** 2048871110006021 **

DR. BROWN

			Billed	Approved
01	Hsp Consultation	March 21, 1990	$145.00	$127.75

Approved amount limited by 5C on back.

Total approved for all services on this claim $127.75
Medicare payment (80 percent of the approved amount) $102.20

We are paying a total of $102.20 to you on the enclosed check. Please cash it as soon as possible. If you have private insurance, it may help with the part Medicare did not pay.

  (You have now met $75.00 of the $75.00 deductible for 1990.)

IMPORTANT: If you do not agree with the amounts approved, you may ask for a review. To do this, write to us before October 27, 1990. (See item 1 on the back.)

DO YOU HAVE A QUESTION ABOUT THIS NOTICE? If you believe Medicare paid for a service you did not receive, or there is an error, contact us immediately.

Participating doctors and suppliers always accept assignment of Medicare claims. See back of this notice for an explanation of assignment. You can get more information by calling the number shown above.

Medicare Claim No. 123456789A

YOUR MEDICARE MEDICAL INSURANCE CLAIMS RECORD

Note: You can use the "Other Remarks" column to keep track of your medical insurance deductible until it's met or for notes about appeals or private supplementary insurance.

Date you mailed claim	Date of service or supply	Doctor or supplier who provided service or supply	Service or supply you received	Charge for service or supply	Date and amount of Medicare payment	Other Remarks

Appendix D: Participating Medicare Providers by State

State	Percentage of doctors who are participating providers
Alabama	75.9
Alaska	38.8
Arizona	41.2
Arkansas	53.1
California	54.0
Colorado	28.1
Connecticut	29.3[1]
Delaware	37.5
District of Columbia	34.4
Florida	32.8
Georgia	49.7
Hawaii	53.7
Idaho	16.0
Illinois	40.0
Indiana	40.0
Iowa	45.3

PARTICIPATING MEDICARE PROVIDERS BY STATE
(continued)

State	Percentage of doctors who are participating providers
Kansas	61.6
Kentucky	50.5
Louisiana	32.6
Maine	51.2
Maryland	42.8
Massachusetts	46.9[2]
Michigan	41.7
Minnesota	25.4
Mississippi	33.4
Missouri	39.6
Montana	21.5
Nebraska	42.5
Nevada	57.0
New Hampshire	28.0
New Jersey	26.0
New Mexico	36.3
New York	29.8
North Carolina	54.2
North Dakota	31.7
Ohio	46.8
Oklahoma	31.6
Oregon	36.9
Pennsylvania	39.0
Rhode Island	58.8[3]
South Carolina	42.1
South Dakota	20.0
Tennessee	57.6
Texas	28.9
Utah	54.7
Vermont	40.5[4]
Virginia	40.9

PARTICIPATING MEDICARE PROVIDERS BY STATE
(continued)

State	Percentage of doctors who are participating providers
Washington	31.4
West Virginia	59.1
Wisconsin	40.0
Wyoming	19.3
All states	40.7

Source: Health Care Financing Administration
Data as of January 1989.

[1] In 1989, Connecticut passed a law prohibiting physicians from charging Medicare patients more than the Medicare-approved amount.

[2] Massachusetts prohibits physicians from charging Medicare patients more than the Medicare-approved amount.

[3] Rhode Island prohibits physicians from collecting excess charges from Medicare patients with incomes of less than $12,000 a year ($15,000 for a couple).

[4] Vermont prohibits physicians from collecting excess fees from Medicare patients with incomes of less than $25,000 a year ($32,000 for a couple). Physicians are allowed to charge more than the Medicare-approved amount for office and home visits.

Further Reading

Aging America: Trends and Projections, 1985–86 edition, Select Committee on Aging, U.S. Senate, 1986.

Bausell, R. Barker, Michael A. Rooney, and Charles B. Inlander. *How to Evaluate and Select a Nursing Home*. Reading, MA: Addison-Wesley, 1988.

The Best Medicine: Organizing Local Health Care Campaigns. Washington D.C.: Villers Foundation (Families, U.S.A.), 1984.

Callahan, Daniel. *Setting Limits: Medical Goals in an Aging Society*. New York: Simon & Schuster, 1987.

Catastrophic Health Insurance: The "Medigap" Crisis. Select Committee on Aging, U.S. House of Representatives, 1986.

Gold, Margaret. *Guide to Housing Alternatives for Older Citizens*. Mount Vernon, NY: Consumers Union, 1985.

The Insurance Dictionary: Life and Health Edition. Chicago, IL: Longman Group, 1985.

Long-term Care for the Elderly: Issues of Need, Access, and Cost. Washington, D.C.: General Accounting Office, 1988.

Medicare and Medicaid Data Book, 1988. Baltimore, MD: Health Care Financing Administration, Office of Research and Demonstrations, 1989.

Medicare Prospective Payment and the American Health System, Report to Congress. Washington, D.C.: Prospective Payments Assessment Commission, 1989.

Nursing Home Ratings 1988. Seattle–King County edition and Snohomish–Skagit and Island Counties edition. Vashon, WA: Washington Nursing Home Rating Service, 1988.

Preventing Medigap Abuse: A Protection Kit for California Seniors. San Francisco: California Department of Insurance, 1988.

198

Rivlin, Alice M., and Joshua M. Wiener. *Caring for the Disabled Elderly: Who Will Pay?* Washington, D.C.: The Brookings Institute, 1988.

Social Security Programs in the United States. Washington, D.C.: Social Security Administration, 1989.

Shelly, Florence D. *When Your Parents Grow Old.* New York: Harper & Row, 1988.

Insurance Terms at a Glance

Accident insurance. Insurance that pays a fixed amount if you are injured in an accident.

Actual charge. The amount a health-care provider charges you for a service. In some cases, the actual charge may be larger than the amount "approved" by Medicare.

Approved charge. The amount Medicare sets as the maximum fee to be charged for a service it covers. This "approved" amount may be the same or less than the actual charge. Under Part B (Medical Insurance), Medicare pays 80 percent of the approved charge. Approved charges are also referred to as "allowable charges" or "reasonable charges."

Assignment. The understanding by which physicians agree to limit their charges to the amounts approved by Medicare. Doctors who accept this agreement to "take assignment" bill Medicare directly for their services. Medicare pays them 80 percent of the approved charge, less any part of your $75 Part-B deductible that has not been met.

Benefits. What Medicare or a private insurance company promises to pay.

Cancelable. A cancelable policy is one that an insurance company has the right to cancel at any time, as opposed to policies that are guaranteed renewable. Generally, companies are required to give you written notice at least 30 days before they cancel.

Carrier. An insurance company hired by the federal government to review and pay Part-B Medicare claims.

Certificate of insurance. Instead of a policy, members of a group insurance plan receive certificates of insurance. (See **Group insurance.**)

Claim. The request for payment sent by you or your health-care provider to a carrier, intermediary, or private insurance company.

Conditionally renewable. The company may cancel a conditionally renewable policy only if it cancels all other policies in its class. A "class" is a group of policies with similar characteristics and may be large or small, depending on how the company has defined it.

Conversion. The right of a policyholder to apply for and receive an individual policy upon termination of group coverage.

Co-payment or co-insurance. A provision requiring that you pay part of the covered expense. The portion you are required to pay is the co-payment or co-insurance.

Custodial care. Care that helps persons with bathing, eating, dressing, taking medications, and other daily activities of life, as opposed to skilled nursing care.

Deductible. An insurance policy may require that you pay a specified amount before the insurance company begins to pay for covered expenses. The specified amount is the deductible. For example, a policy might pay for prescription drugs only after you have paid more than $150 a year in such expenses. The $150 is the deductible.

Dread-disease insurance. Insurance that pays you only if you need treatment for a particular disease, such as cancer. These policies will not pay you if you need treatment for any other reason, nor will they pay if you have already been diagnosed or treated for the disease they cover.

Effective date. The date your insurance coverage begins.

Enrollment period. The specified time during which you can sign up for Medicare. Older Americans who do not qualify for Social Security retirement benefits are permitted to sign up for Medicare only during an enrollment period. The "initial enrollment period" begins three months before the first day of the month in which you have your 65th birthday and extends for seven months. There is also a "general enrollment period" from January 1 to March 31 of each year. You may have to pay more for Medicare coverage if you fail to sign up during your initial enrollment period.

Excess charge: The difference between a doctor's or other health-care provider's actual charge and the Medicare-approved charge.

Explanation of Medical Benefits (EOMB). A notice from the Medicare insurance carrier informing you how much it has paid for a service covered by Medicare Part B (Medical Insurance). For assigned services—those approved by Medicare—the carrier pays the doctor or other provider directly. For unassigned services, the carrier pays you, and you are responsible for paying the provider.

Grace period. The period of time a policy will remain in effect after a payment is due but has not been paid. A 30-day grace period means that the policy will be canceled if you do not make payment within 30 days of the due date.

Group insurance. Insurance provided by prior agreement to a specific group of people—for example, employees of a particular business or members of an association. Technically, the company issues a "master policy" to the business or association. Covered employees or members are issued "certificates of insurance" rather than policies.

Guaranteed renewable. A policy that is guaranteed renewable cannot be canceled by the company as long as you pay your premium. At the end of a policy term—for example, a year—the company must renew your policy on the same terms and conditions, although it may increase the premium.

Health Care Financing Administration (HCFA). The federal agency under the U.S. Department of Health and Human Services that is responsible for overseeing the Medicare program.

Health Maintenance Organization (HMO). An HMO provides health care to its members and charges them a fixed amount per month. Some HMOs accept seniors enrolled in Medicare. These HMOs provide all of the services covered by Medicare and charge a fixed amount instead of the normal deductibles, co-payments, and excess charges. Some HMOs also cover services that are not covered by Medicare, such as eyeglasses and prescription drugs.

Hearing officer. A person hired by the Medicare insurance carrier to hear and decide appeals.

Hospital indemnity insurance. Insurance that pays you a fixed amount for each day you are hospitalized. While relatively inexpensive, these policies are not designed to keep up with the rising cost of hospital care, nor will they pay for non-hospital-related expenses.

Insured. The person covered by an insurance policy.

Inpatient. In general, a patient who is admitted to a hospital or skilled nursing facility and stays overnight during his or her treatment.

Intermediary. An insurance company hired by the federal government to review and pay Medicare Part-A (Hospital Insurance) claims.

Intermediate nursing facility. A facility that is staffed and equipped to provide less intensive care than a skilled nursing facility. Nursing and rehabilitative care are still regularly provided by licensed professionals, but on less than a daily basis.

Lifetime reserve day. If you are hospitalized for longer than 90 days during a spell of illness, Medicare will pay for up to 60 additional days of care. Each of those 60 days is called a reserve day and can be used only once during your lifetime.

Medicare. The federal program that pays for some of the health-care expenses for people (1) over age 65, (2) who have been disabled for at least 24 months, or (3) with serious kidney disease. Medicare is divided into two parts: Part A (Hospital Insurance) and Part B (Medical Insurance).

Medicaid. The government program that pays for some of the health-care expenses for low-income persons, regardless of age. Each state operates its own Medicaid program under certain general rules established by the federal government.

Medically needy. People with incomes that are above the poverty line but who need financial assistance because of large medical expenses are medically needy. Thirty-five states have expanded their Medicaid programs to cover people who are medically needy.

Medical-surgical insurance. Insurance that pays a fixed amount for each covered medical service you receive. These policies generally duplicate Medicare Part-B coverage and are not designed to keep up with inflation.

Medicare benefit notice. A notice from a Medicare insurance intermediary informing you how much it has paid a doctor or other health-care provider for a service covered by Medicare Part A (Hospital Insurance).

Medicare supplement insurance (or Medigap insurance). Insurance designed specifically to provide additional coverage for people on Medicare. Such policies typically pay for Medicare deductibles and co-payments. Some pay for a few services that are not covered by Medicare, such as eyeglasses or prescription drugs.

Outpatient. A patient who receives treatment in a hospital, clinic, emergency room, or skilled nursing facility but does not stay overnight there.

Part A. The part of Medicare that covers inpatient hospital care, care in a skilled nursing facility, hospice care, and short-term home health care.

Part B. The part of Medicare that covers doctors' services, outpatient hospital care, lab tests, X rays, and durable medical equipment.

Participating physicians. Doctors who will accept assignment—the Medicare-approved payment—for all of the services they provide to Medicare patients.

Policy. The contract between you and the insurance company.

Pre-existing condition. A medical condition that you knew existed before the effective date of your insurance.

Premium. The amount of money you must pay to keep an insurance policy in effect.

Proof of loss. The information you need to send an insurance company before it will pay for covered expenses. This information may include such documents as doctors' bills and Explanations of Medical Benefits from Medicare (EOMBs).

Skilled nursing facility. A facility that is specially staffed and equipped to provide intensive nursing and rehabilitative care to patients. Care is provided by licensed nurses or licensed therapists under the supervision of a doctor.

Social Security law judge. A person employed by the Social Security Administration to hear and decide Medicare appeals.

Spell of illness. Under Medicare Part A (Hospital Insurance), a spell of illness begins on the first day you are admitted as an inpatient to a hospital or skilled nursing facility and extends until you have been out of the hospital or skilled nursing facility for 60 consecutive days. For each spell of illness, Medicare Part A will cover up to 90 days of hospital care and 100 days of care in a skilled nursing facility.

Spending down. The process of depleting your assets and income until you are poor enough to qualify for Medicaid.

Waiver of liability. A provision that excuses you from paying insurance premiums under certain conditions—for example, if you are admitted to a hospital or nursing home.

Index